I0704875

Table of Contents

Introduction 5

Understanding the Lymphatic System 11

The Impact of Toxins on Weight and Health 19

Breaking Free From Sugar 43

Understanding Gut Health and Detoxification 47

Nutrition for Detox and Weight Loss 65

Nourishing Recipes 73

Hydration and Clean Water 101

Stimulating the Lymphatic System 109

Herbs and Adaptogens for Detox 125

Managing Stress and Emotional Toxins 133

Healing Inflammation With Electrons from the Earth 137

The Power of Intention in Detox and Healing 143

Embracing a Lifestyle of Balance and Wellness 149

Introduction

Our bodies are constantly exposed to a wide variety of toxins, from environmental pollutants to chemicals in food, water, and everyday products. Over time, these toxins accumulate in our bodies, straining our natural detoxification systems and making it harder for us to maintain optimal health and weight. Detoxification, therefore, is not just a trendy concept—it's an essential practice for restoring balance, boosting vitality, and achieving healthy, sustainable weight loss. By understanding how detoxification works, and its connection to the lymphatic system, we can unlock a natural pathway to wellness and weight management.

Detoxification, or "detox," is the body's process of eliminating waste products and toxins that accumulate through daily life. Our bodies are naturally designed to detoxify. Major organs like the liver, kidneys, lungs, skin, and intestines work continuously to filter and excrete harmful substances. However, due to modern lifestyles—characterized by processed foods, sedentary habits, environmental toxins, and chronic stress—our bodies often become overwhelmed, and our detox pathways may not function as efficiently as they should.

Engaging in a detox involves specific practices and dietary strategies that support and enhance these natural detoxification pathways, helping the body eliminate built-up waste, restore metabolic balance, and reduce the burden on vital organs. For those aiming to lose weight, detoxification can play an important role by improving metabolic efficiency, reducing inflammation, and encouraging the release of stored toxins from fat cells.

Toxins are often stored in fat tissue to protect the body from their harmful effects. When the body is exposed to an excess of toxins, it may increase fat storage to contain these substances. A well-planned detox encourages the breakdown of fat tissue, releasing these stored toxins for excretion. This process not only aids in weight loss but also helps reduce the toxic burden on the body.

Many toxins contribute to low-level, chronic inflammation, which can hinder weight loss and compromise immune function. Inflammation disrupts metabolic processes and promotes the release of cortisol, a stress hormone that encourages fat storage, especially around the abdomen. Detoxification reduces inflammation, improving metabolic efficiency and supporting the body's ability to burn fat.

When the liver and other detox organs are overburdened, metabolism slows down, making it harder to burn calories efficiently. By supporting these organs, detoxification can enhance metabolic function, leading to better energy balance, improved digestion, and more effective weight management.

One of the lesser-known, yet incredibly important components of detoxification and weight loss is the lymphatic system. The lymphatic system is a network of vessels, nodes, and organs that circulates lymph fluid—a clear, watery substance containing white blood cells—throughout the body. It plays a central role in immune defense, fluid balance, and, importantly, waste removal.

Here's how the lymphatic system supports detox and weight loss:

Clearing Toxins and Waste The lymphatic system collects and transports waste products, toxins, and excess fluids from tissues back to the bloodstream, where they can be processed and eliminated. A healthy lymphatic flow is essential for removing these wastes efficiently. When the lymphatic system becomes sluggish or congested, toxins build up, and fat storage may increase as the body tries to protect itself.

Regulating Fluid Balance Proper lymphatic function prevents fluid retention and bloating, common issues that can make us feel heavier and look puffier. By promoting lymphatic drainage, detoxification helps to reduce fluid buildup, improving both comfort and appearance.

Supporting Immune Health The lymphatic system is a key player in immune function, carrying white blood cells and filtering pathogens through lymph nodes. Detox practices that support the lymphatic system can enhance immunity, which is crucial for overall health and energy levels, making it easier to stay active and motivated on a weight loss journey.

The primary goals of a detox cleanse are not only to support weight loss but also to improve energy levels, boost immune function, and restore the body's natural vitality.

A well-designed detox targets stubborn fat deposits and helps the body to release and process stored toxins. By addressing factors that contribute to weight gain—like inflammation, sluggish metabolism, and hormonal imbalances—a detox can facilitate sustainable weight loss. This isn't about crash dieting or rapid weight loss but rather a gentle, holistic approach that encourages the body to naturally let go of excess weight.

A detox that supports the lymphatic system and other detox organs also strengthens the immune system. When toxins are effectively cleared, the immune system operates more efficiently, protecting the body from infections and reducing inflammation. This increased immunity not only contributes to weight loss by reducing stress and inflammation but also supports overall health, making it easier to resist illness and bounce back from daily stressors.

As the body clears out toxins and improves metabolic function, you're likely to experience a noticeable increase in energy levels. Detoxification reduces the strain on the liver, kidneys, and digestive system, freeing up energy that was previously used for processing waste. Many people report feeling lighter, more energetic, and mentally clearer during and after a detox cleanse, making it easier to maintain healthy lifestyle choices and pursue fitness goals.

Detoxification is not just a short-term strategy but a pathway to sustainable wellness. By focusing on lymphatic health, reducing toxin exposure, and supporting the body's natural detox pathways, a detox cleanse lays the foundation for a healthier, more vibrant life. It's an opportunity to reset not only your physical health but also your mindset and habits around food, hydration, movement, and self-care.

Whether you're seeking weight loss, better energy, or simply a way to feel healthier, embracing detox as a lifestyle approach can help you achieve lasting wellness. By taking steps to support detoxification regularly, you're empowering your body to work at its best, clearing out what no longer serves you, and creating space for renewed health and vitality.

Understanding the Lymphatic System

The lymphatic system works alongside the circulatory system to transport a clear fluid called lymph, which carries waste products, toxins, and immune cells throughout the body. Lymph fluid is rich in white blood cells (especially lymphocytes), which are essential for fighting off infections and protecting the body from harmful invaders (your immune system).

Unlike the circulatory system, which has the heart as a pump, the *lymphatic system lacks a central pump of its own*. This creates unique challenges in keeping lymph fluid moving, making it crucial to support this system through lifestyle practices and physical movement.

As lymph fluid circulates through the body, it gathers cellular waste, bacteria, viruses, and other toxins. It is then transported to lymph nodes, which filter out harmful substances before allowing the fluid to re-enter the bloodstream.

In addition to filtering waste, the lymphatic system is also responsible for absorbing fats and fat-soluble nutrients from the digestive tract and transporting them to the bloodstream. This function contributes to the body's overall energy balance and nutrient distribution, which are essential for maintaining metabolic health.

The lymphatic system is made up of several interconnected structures that each play a unique role:

Lymph Vessels These thin-walled vessels are spread throughout the body and act as the transport network for lymph fluid. Lymph vessels are similar to veins in the circulatory system but are much finer. They carry lymph fluid from tissues back toward the larger lymph nodes and eventually to the bloodstream.

Lymph Nodes Small, bean-shaped structures located along the lymph vessels, lymph nodes act as filtration points where immune cells (such as lymphocytes and macrophages) capture and destroy pathogens, toxins, and cellular waste. They are concentrated in areas such as the neck, armpits, chest, abdomen, and groin. When the body is fighting an infection, lymph nodes may swell as they filter and trap harmful agents.

Thymus Located behind the breastbone, the thymus is where T-cells (a type of white blood cell) mature. T-cells play a crucial role in immune response, recognizing and targeting pathogens and abnormal cells.

Spleen The largest organ in the lymphatic system, the spleen is responsible for filtering blood, recycling old red blood cells, and storing white blood cells and platelets. It also helps combat certain kinds of bacteria that cause pneumonia and meningitis.

Tonsils and Adenoids Located in the throat, the tonsils and adenoids are lymphoid tissues that act as the first line of defense against inhaled or ingested pathogens. They play an important role in developing immune responses, particularly in childhood.

Bone Marrow Though not directly part of the lymphatic "transport" system, bone marrow is crucial for producing the white blood cells that populate the lymphatic system and defend the body against infections.

Peyer's Patches These are small lymphoid tissues found in the small intestine, which help protect the body from ingested pathogens and contribute to gut immunity.

Given that the lymphatic system lacks a pumping mechanism of its own, lymph flow depends on a combination of factors:

Muscle Movement Physical movement and muscle contractions help compress lymph vessels, pushing lymph fluid through the system. This is one of the reasons exercise feels so good, but also massage, hydrotherapy, and skin brushing all have an invigorating effect on how we feel.

Breathing Deep breathing, especially from the diaphragm, creates pressure changes in the chest that promote lymph flow.

Gravity Elevating certain areas of the body, like the legs, can help encourage lymph drainage.

Without a dedicated pump, the lymphatic system can easily become stagnant if these factors aren't regularly engaged. A lack of movement, shallow breathing, or a sedentary lifestyle can all contribute to a sluggish lymphatic system, which makes it more challenging for the body to effectively remove waste and toxins.

When the lymphatic system isn't working optimally, toxins and waste can accumulate, leading to a variety of symptoms. Signs of a sluggish lymphatic system may include:

Swelling and Puffiness The most common sign of lymphatic congestion is swelling, particularly in the extremities like the ankles, fingers, and under the eyes. This fluid retention can give a feeling of heaviness or bloating.

Frequent Infections A compromised lymphatic system may lead to a weakened immune response, making the body more susceptible to infections, colds, and flu.

Skin Issues Acne, rashes, eczema, and other skin problems may arise as the body tries to expel toxins through the skin when lymph flow is slow.

Fatigue A sluggish lymphatic system can cause feelings of tiredness and lethargy as the body becomes overwhelmed by accumulated waste and lacks efficient detoxification.

Muscle and Joint Pain When toxins accumulate in tissues, it can cause inflammation that leads to muscle aches, joint stiffness, and general discomfort.

Brain Fog The build-up of toxins can affect mental clarity, causing symptoms such as brain fog, poor concentration, and memory issues.

Cellulite and Weight Gain Poor lymphatic flow can lead to a build-up of toxins and fats in the tissues, contributing to stubborn weight gain, water retention, and the appearance of cellulite.

Digestive Issues Digestive discomfort, such as bloating and constipation, can indicate poor lymphatic drainage, particularly if the digestive tract is not adequately absorbing and transporting nutrients.

Cold Hands and Feet Poor lymphatic circulation can contribute to poor blood circulation, resulting in cold hands and feet. If your lymphatic system is sluggish, blood flow may be compromised, making extremities feel cold more frequently, even in warm environments.

WHY SUPPORTING THE LYMPHATIC SYSTEM IS ESSENTIAL FOR DETOX AND WEIGHT LOSS

The lymphatic system is intricately linked to the body's ability to detoxify, maintain a healthy weight, and keep the immune system functioning optimally. When lymph flow is sluggish, the body's natural detox processes are impaired, leading to toxin build-up, inflammation, and compromised immune defense. For those seeking to lose weight, addressing lymphatic health is particularly important. As the lymphatic system removes waste products from the body, it helps reduce fluid retention and bloating, making you feel lighter and more energized.

Improving lymphatic flow through diet, exercise, and lifestyle practices (such as dry brushing, lymphatic massage, or even regular movement and deep breathing) can support the body's natural detoxification pathways, aiding in weight management, enhancing skin appearance, and boosting energy levels.

By maintaining a healthy lymphatic system, you empower your body's natural ability to clear waste, reduce inflammation, and create an internal environment conducive to long-term wellness and vitality.

The Impact of Toxins on Weight and Health

Many people associate toxins with harmful chemicals in the environment, but in reality, toxins are everywhere. They enter our bodies through food, water, lifestyle habits, and even from everyday household products. Over time, the accumulation of these toxins can disrupt our body's natural processes, leading to health issues, weight gain, and difficulty in shedding pounds. Understanding the sources of toxins and how they impact our weight and overall health is crucial for anyone pursuing a detox cleanse.

Toxins can enter our bodies in various ways. Here's a look at some of the primary sources:

Food Sadly, our diet is one of the largest contributors to toxin exposure. Processed foods are often filled with artificial Ingredients, preservatives, and additives to enhance flavor, texture, or shelf life. Many of these substances are foreign to our bodies, making it difficult to break them down or eliminate them efficiently.

Pesticides Modern agriculture relies heavily on pesticides to increase crop yields and protect plants from pests. However, these chemicals leave residues on fruits and vegetables that can accumulate in the human body over time, contributing to our overall "toxic load." Let's look closer at some of the most common pesticides, their potential health risks, and ways to minimize exposure.

When we consume pesticide residues, they enter our system and may be processed by the liver and kidneys. However, due to the synthetic nature of many pesticides, the body can have difficulty breaking them down completely, leading to an accumulation of toxins over time. These chemicals can interact with various bodily systems, potentially causing both acute and long-term health effects.

Glyphosate Glyphosate is a widely used herbicide, particularly on crops like wheat, corn and soy. It is commonly used in non-organic farming to control weeds. Studies have linked glyphosate to hormone disruption, liver and kidney toxicity, and even certain cancers, such as non-Hodgkin's lymphoma. Glyphosate has also been shown to interfere with the gut microbiome, potentially impacting digestion and immunity.

Organophosphates *Originally developed as nerve agents,* organophosphates are a class of pesticides that are now used on many fruits and vegetables, including apples, grapes, and bell peppers. These chemicals are known to disrupt the nervous system by inhibiting certain enzymes essential for nerve function. This disruption has been associated with developmental issues in children, including impacts on cognitive and behavioral functions, as well as an increased risk of neurological diseases later in life.

Atrazine Atrazine is a herbicide primarily used on corn but is also found in other crop applications. Atrazine is known to disrupt endocrine function, affecting hormone balance, and has been linked to reproductive and developmental issues. Studies have shown that atrazine exposure can lead to lower fertility rates and hormonal imbalances, with some research even suggesting possible links to birth defects.

Pesticides can have a wide range of effects on the body. Here are some of the most significant health risks associated with long-term exposure to these chemicals:

Endocrine Disruption Many pesticides act as endocrine disruptors, which means they can mimic or interfere with hormones, the body's chemical messengers. This interference can affect reproductive health, weight gain, thyroid function, and may lead to conditions like polycystic ovary syndrome (PCOS) and hormone-sensitive cancers. Children are especially vulnerable to endocrine disruption as their hormonal systems are still developing.

Immune System Suppression Pesticides may weaken the immune system by increasing oxidative stress and inflammation in the body. This suppression makes it harder for the immune system to fight infections, recover from illnesses, and can increase susceptibility to autoimmune disorders.

Increased Inflammatory Response Exposure to pesticides can cause inflammation, particularly in the liver and lungs, as the body works to detoxify these chemicals. Chronic inflammation is linked to a range of diseases, including cardiovascular disease, diabetes, and respiratory conditions. Inflammation due to pesticide exposure can also strain the liver, one of the body's primary detox organs, reducing its ability to filter out other toxins effectively.

While it's challenging to avoid pesticides entirely, there are several effective strategies for minimizing your intake and protecting your health:

Choose Organic When Possible Organic produce is grown without synthetic pesticides, which significantly reduces your exposure to these chemicals. Although organic options can sometimes be more expensive, prioritizing organic versions of the most contaminated foods (known as the "Dirty Dozen") can make a big difference.

Understanding the Dirty Dozen and Clean Fifteen Each year, the Environmental Working Group (EWG) releases the Dirty Dozen list, highlighting fruits and vegetables with the highest levels of pesticide residues. Some commonly included items are strawberries, spinach, bell peppers, grapes, blueberries, green beans, and apples. By choosing organic versions of these items, you can reduce your pesticide exposure considerably.

The EWG also publishes a Clean Fifteen list, which includes produce with the lowest pesticide residues. If you're on a budget, you may want to prioritize organic options for the Dirty Dozen while choosing conventional versions of Clean Fifteen items, like avocados and sweet corn.

Using a Produce Wash Even with non-organic produce, you can reduce pesticide residues by using a produce wash. Soaking fruits and vegetables in a mixture of water and vinegar (1:3 ratio) for 10-15 minutes and rinsing thoroughly can help to remove surface pesticides, though it may not eliminate all residues that have penetrated the skin.

Peeling and Scrubbing For certain produce, peeling the skin can reduce pesticide exposure since residues often concentrate on the surface. However, some fruits and vegetables have beneficial nutrients in their skin, so weigh the pros and cons based on the produce. Scrubbing firm produce like potatoes, cucumbers, and carrots with a vegetable brush can also help remove residues.

While reducing pesticide exposure is essential, it's also helpful to support your body's natural detoxification processes to handle any remaining exposure:

Increase Antioxidant-Rich Foods Foods high in antioxidants, such as berries, leafy greens, and cruciferous vegetables, help the body fight oxidative stress caused by pesticides and other toxins. Antioxidants can protect cells from damage and support the liver's ability to process and eliminate chemicals.

Support the Liver with Detoxifying Herbs Herbs like milk thistle, dandelion root, and turmeric have been shown to support liver function, helping the body process and eliminate toxins more effectively. These can be taken as supplements or added to your diet in teas and meals.

Focus on Fiber-Rich Foods Fiber binds to toxins in the digestive tract and helps carry them out of the body. Increasing fiber intake through foods like oats, chia seeds, and legumes aids digestion and reduces the time toxins spend in your system, minimizing reabsorption.

In conclusion, while pesticides help in food production, they come with potential health risks due to the toxic residues left on produce. By making informed choices, such as prioritizing organic foods, using effective washing techniques, and supporting your body's detox mechanisms, you can reduce your pesticide exposure and protect your health. Integrating these practices into your lifestyle can help manage the toxic load and support a clean, balanced, and resilient body over the long term.

ADDITIVES AND PRESERVATIVES IN PROCESSED FOODS

In addition to pesticides, many processed foods also contain additives and preservatives—substances that enhance flavor, color, or shelf life but may have adverse effects on health. Regular consumption of these compounds has been linked to hormonal disruption, metabolic disturbances, immune suppression, and an increased risk of inflammation-related diseases. Let's explore some common additives and preservatives, their potential health risks, and steps to minimize exposure.

Red 40 (FD&C Red 40) Red 40 is a synthetic dye derived from petroleum. It is commonly found in soft drinks, candies, snack foods, and baked goods. Red 40 has been associated with hyperactivity in children and can trigger migraines in both children and adults. Some research suggests it may also cause DNA damage, potentially leading to cellular changes over time. Red 40 is banned in several countries, including Norway, Switzerland, and Japan, due to these concerns. While permitted in the EU, it must carry a warning label indicating possible behavioral effects in children.

To protect yourself, look for natural alternatives to artificially colored foods, such as snacks made with real fruit or vegetables, which are often colored with turmeric, beets, or paprika.

BHA and BHT (Butylated Hydroxyanisole and Butylated Hydroxytoluene) These synthetic antioxidants are added to prevent oils and fats from going rancid. They are commonly found in processed snacks, cereals, and chewing gum. BHA and BHT are suspected endocrine disruptors, meaning they may interfere with hormone function and could potentially impact reproductive health. Some studies have shown that they can affect thyroid function and estrogen levels. Additionally, BHA is classified as a possible carcinogen by the International Agency for Research on Cancer (IARC).

To avoid BHA and BHT, check food labels and choose products without BHA and BHT. Opt for foods that use natural antioxidants like vitamin E or rosemary extract to preserve freshness.

Sodium Benzoate Sodium benzoate is a preservative commonly found in acidic foods like sodas, salad dressings, fruit juices, and condiments. When combined with vitamin C, sodium benzoate can form benzene, a known carcinogen linked to leukemia and other blood disorders. Long-term exposure has also been associated with increased oxidative stress and potential damage to cellular structures.

By choosing fresh, whole foods over processed ones, and beverages and condiments labeled "preservative-free," or making homemade salad dressings and sauces you can avoid this additive.

Nitrates and Nitrites These compounds are used to cure and preserve meats like bacon, sausages, and deli products. They give processed meats their characteristic pink color and enhance flavor.

Nitrates and nitrites can form **nitrosamines** when exposed to high temperatures (such as during frying), which are known carcinogens linked to gastrointestinal cancers and other inflammatory diseases. These compounds have also been linked to vascular inflammation, which can contribute to cardiovascular problems.

Avoid fried meats and highly-processed meats, instead, choose nitrate-free and nitrite-free meat options when possible. Look for "uncured" or "no nitrates added" labels, and consider plant-based alternatives for processed meats.

HEALTH RISKS OF ADDITIVES AND PRESERVATIVES

Endocrine Disruption Many additives, such as BHA, BHT, and certain food dyes, act as endocrine disruptors, meaning they can interfere with hormone production, signaling, and balance. These disruptions may lead to weight gain, thyroid issues, reproductive problems, and developmental concerns, especially in children.

Gut Health and Dysbiosis Certain preservatives can negatively impact the gut microbiome, reducing the number of beneficial bacteria and promoting the growth of harmful ones. This imbalance, known as dysbiosis, is linked to digestive issues, immune system weakness, and even mood disorders due to the gut-brain connection. Gut health is critical to overall wellness, and disturbances in microbial balance can increase inflammation and contribute to chronic health conditions.

Immune System Suppression Synthetic preservatives and additives can strain the immune system by increasing oxidative stress and inflammation. Over time, this exposure can reduce the immune system's efficiency, making it harder for the body to fight infections and recover from illness.

Increased Inflammatory Response Additives and preservatives often trigger inflammatory responses in the body, particularly affecting the liver, where these substances are metabolized. Chronic inflammation has been linked to a wide range of conditions, from arthritis and cardiovascular disease to metabolic syndrome and cancer.

In addition to additives and preservatives, certain cooking oils can also contribute to inflammation in the body. High-omega-6 oils and refined oils are particularly problematic, as they create an imbalance in the body's fatty acid profile and introduce harmful compounds when heated to high temperatures.

Vegetable Oil Vegetable oil is usually a blend of oils, such as soybean, corn, and canola oil, that are highly processed to be shelf-stable. Vegetable oil is rich in omega-6 fatty acids, which, when consumed in excess, can promote inflammation. This is particularly problematic if your diet lacks sufficient omega-3s to counterbalance the effect. Excess omega-6 intake is associated with chronic inflammation, cardiovascular disease, and metabolic issues.

The better option is to use healthier alternatives, such as extra virgin olive oil, avocado oil, or coconut oil, which have more favorable fatty acid profiles and lower omega-6 levels.

Canola Oil Canola oil has a relatively balanced omega-6 to omega-3 ratio, but it is typically highly refined, which strips it of beneficial nutrients and can introduce trans fats. Due to high-temperature processing, refined canola oil may contain small amounts of trans fats, which raise LDL cholesterol and increase the risk of heart disease. The refining process can also reduce antioxidant content, diminishing its health benefits.

If you choose canola oil, look for cold-pressed or minimally refined options. Otherwise, opt for oils like olive or avocado oil, which retain more nutrients and are less inflammatory.

Soybean Oil Soybean oil is widely used in processed foods and restaurant cooking. It's inexpensive and has a long shelf life, making it a popular choice. Soybean oil is high in omega-6 fatty acids and has been linked to inflammation, obesity, and metabolic dysfunction. Research suggests that diets high in soybean oil may disrupt glucose metabolism and negatively impact heart health.

It's best to limit processed and restaurant foods that commonly use soybean oil, and consider preparing meals at home using healthier oils.

HEALTH RISKS OF INFLAMMATORY COOKING OILS

Chronic Inflammation A diet high in omega-6 fatty acids and low in omega-3s can create a pro-inflammatory state, contributing to a range of chronic diseases, including arthritis, heart disease, and inflammatory bowel disease. The imbalance in fatty acid intake is a significant driver of systemic inflammation.

Increased Risk of Heart Disease Refined oils often undergo processing that introduces trans fats, which are known to raise LDL ("bad") cholesterol and lower HDL ("good") cholesterol. This increases the risk of heart disease and is a leading cause of cardiovascular issues.

Oxidative Stress and Free Radical Formation When oils are heated to high temperatures, they can oxidize and produce **free radicals**—unstable molecules that cause oxidative stress, damaging cells and contributing to aging, inflammation, and disease. This is particularly common with unstable oils like vegetable and soybean oil.

CHOOSING HEALTHIER ALTERNATIVES

Anti-Inflammatory Oils Use oils that are less processed and retain their nutrient profiles, such as extra virgin olive oil, avocado oil, and coconut oil. These oils have lower omega-6 levels and a stable fat profile, making them ideal for cooking at moderate temperatures.

Cooking Techniques Avoid high-heat methods with unstable oils. Opt for steaming, baking, or sautéing at low to medium heat. This reduces the need for oils that are prone to oxidation at high temperatures.

Read Labels Carefully Look for foods that are free from artificial colors, preservatives, and inflammatory oils. Many brands now offer options without these additives, and cooking at home with whole foods can help you avoid them altogether.

By being mindful of the additives, preservatives, and oils in our food, we can make healthier choices that reduce our toxic load, support our hormone balance, and promote overall well-being. Integrating these practices into our daily lives helps build a foundation for long-term health and vitality.

TOXINS IN THE WATER

Water is essential for detoxification, but many tap and even some bottled waters contain impurities that burden the body, especially if they are labeled as being from a "municipal source," which means they are essentially tap water sold in bottles.

Hormone Disruptors Synthetic hormones, such as those from birth control pills, are increasingly present in our water supplies due to wastewater contamination. Even in trace amounts, these hormone disruptors can interfere with our body's natural hormonal balance, affecting functions like metabolism, mood, and reproductive health. When we consume water containing residual synthetic hormones, our bodies—especially the lymphatic system—must work harder to filter these foreign compounds, increasing the toxic load. Over time, this can lead to hormonal imbalances and added stress on both the endocrine and lymphatic systems.

Pharmaceutical Residues Traces of pharmaceuticals, including antibiotics, anti-anxiety medications, and pain relievers, have been detected in drinking water sources worldwide. Although these drugs are present in minute amounts, the effects of long-term, low-level exposure are not yet fully understood. Accumulation of pharmaceutical residues over time may contribute to several health risks, including antibiotic resistance, hormonal disruptions, and even heightened allergic sensitivities in certain individuals. These contaminants can place additional stress on the immune system and increase the workload of the lymphatic system, which must work harder to filter out these foreign substances.

Chemical Leaching from Plastics Plastic bottles and containers often contain chemicals like BPA (bisphenol A) and other endocrine disruptors, which can leach into water, especially when exposed to heat. This leaching process accelerates when plastic bottles are left in warm environments, such as in a car on a hot day. Regular consumption of water contaminated with these chemicals may disrupt hormonal balance, lead to immune stress, and promote inflammation. The lymphatic system, which plays a key role in removing toxins, must handle the additional burden of filtering these synthetic chemicals, further stressing the body's detoxification pathways.

Heavy Metals Lead, mercury, and arsenic can leach into water supplies from pipes, industrial runoff, or natural deposits, and are difficult for the body to process. These heavy metals are toxic and can disrupt hormones, immune function, and cellular repair.

Chlorine and Fluoride: Added to municipal water supplies to disinfect and prevent tooth decay, these chemicals can affect thyroid function and disrupt the gut microbiome.

TOXINS IN FOOD STORAGE CONTAINERS

The containers we use to store and heat our food can introduce toxins into our diet, especially if made of plastic or aluminum.

Plastic Containers Plastics, especially when heated, can leach chemicals like BPA (bisphenol A) and phthalates into food. These chemicals are endocrine disruptors, meaning they interfere with hormones that regulate metabolism, appetite, and fat storage.

Aluminum Foil and Cans Aluminum can leach into food, particularly when heated or in contact with acidic foods. Excessive aluminum exposure has been linked to neurotoxicity and metabolic disruptions.

LIFESTYLE FACTORS THAT AFFECT TOXIN BUILD-UP

Our habits, relationships, and emotional well-being also influence toxin build-up in our bodies.

Stress Chronic stress leads to the release of cortisol, a hormone that, in excess, promotes fat storage (especially around the abdomen) and disrupts blood sugar levels. Stress also weakens the immune system, making it harder for the body to defend itself against toxins.

Toxic Relationships Negative relationships and environments increase stress and create emotional toxins, leading to the release of stress hormones. Persistent exposure to these stressors can impact physical health by promoting inflammation and compromising the body's ability to detoxify.

Lack of Sleep Sleep is essential for cellular repair and detoxification. Without adequate rest, the body can't effectively eliminate waste products or regulate hormones, resulting in increased susceptibility to toxin build-up.

Environmental Toxins The air we breathe and the products we use daily can expose us to a wide range of chemicals.

Air Pollutants Particulate matter from vehicle emissions, factories, and indoor pollutants can carry toxins directly into our respiratory system, where they enter the bloodstream and contribute to inflammation and oxidative stress.

Household Chemicals Cleaning products, air fresheners, and personal care items often contain chemicals that are absorbed through the skin or inhaled. Many of these chemicals are known endocrine disruptors that can affect hormone balance and metabolic health.

HOW TOXINS INTERFERE WITH WEIGHT LOSS

With so many potential sources of toxins in daily life, it's important to understand how these substances can derail weight loss efforts and impact overall health.

Disrupting Metabolism Toxins, particularly endocrine disruptors like BPA, phthalates, and pesticides, interfere with the body's hormonal balance. Hormones are chemical messengers that regulate metabolism, appetite, and energy storage. When toxins disrupt these hormones, the body may struggle to burn calories efficiently or may increase fat storage as a protective mechanism.

Additionally, some toxins accumulate in fat cells. When the body can't immediately eliminate a toxin, it may store it in fat tissue to prevent harm to vital organs. Unfortunately, this can make fat loss more challenging, as breaking down fat cells releases these stored toxins back into circulation, potentially overwhelming the body's detox pathways.

Hormone Imbalance Toxins can mimic or block natural hormones, leading to imbalances that affect weight, mood, and energy. For instance:

Estrogen Mimicker Chemicals like bisphenol A (BPA) and bisphenol S (BPS) mimic estrogen, leading to estrogen dominance, which is associated with weight gain, particularly around the hips and thighs. Plastic bottles, thermal receipt paper, and take-out food packaging are some of the most potent sources of BPA we encounter on a daily basis, which are absorbed through the skin and have been linked to cancer, obesity, and attention problems.

If you work with thermal receipt paper, wear gloves or food-grade silicone tips while working. Don't place your hands in your mouth or eyes after handling receipts, and be careful about washing your hands often with soap and water, especially before lunch breaks.

Thyroid Disruption The thyroid gland regulates metabolism, and certain toxins like fluoride, chlorine, and heavy metals can interfere with thyroid function, slowing down metabolic rate and making weight loss harder.

Compromising Immune Response The immune system plays a critical role in eliminating toxins. When toxins accumulate, they can weaken immune function, making it harder for the body to fend off infections and inflammation. Chronic, low-level inflammation is particularly problematic because it promotes insulin resistance (a precursor to diabetes) and increases fat storage.

Given the many ways toxins interfere with metabolism, hormone balance, and immunity, detoxification becomes essential for weight loss and overall wellness. Detox practices can help to:

Flush Out Stored Toxins Reducing the toxic load by minimizing exposure and actively supporting the body's detoxification pathways allows the body to release stored toxins, especially those accumulated in fat cells.

Reduce Inflammation Detoxing helps the body reduce chronic inflammation, which in turn improves hormone sensitivity, reduces fat storage, and enhances metabolic function.

Support Hormonal Balance By minimizing exposure to endocrine disruptors and using practices that enhance natural detox, the body can rebalance its hormones, making it easier to regulate weight, mood, and energy.

Boost Immunity A healthy detox system, with a well-functioning liver, lymphatic system, and kidneys, supports immunity and aids in clearing out waste effectively. When the immune system is strong, the body can better protect itself against toxins, pathogens, and disease.

Detoxing involves more than simply cleansing the digestive system. It requires a holistic approach to reduce toxin exposure, promote a supportive environment, and empower the body to manage its detox pathways. This approach allows the body to work at its best, balancing metabolism, reducing inflammation, and achieving sustainable weight loss in a way that feels natural and energizing.

Breaking Free From Sugar

Many packaged foods contain high amounts of refined sugars or artificial sweeteners, which can disrupt gut health, contribute to inflammation, and lead to blood sugar imbalances—all of which hinder weight loss.

While sugar may provide a quick burst of energy and pleasure, its impacts on health are far from sweet. Overconsumption of sugar has been linked to a range of harmful effects on the body, affecting everything from metabolic health to immune function. By understanding the toxic effects of sugar, we can make more conscious choices to protect our bodies from its damaging influence.

When we consume sugar, it triggers a powerful response in our brain's reward system, releasing dopamine, a "feel-good" chemical associated with pleasure. However, this dopamine release is part of what makes sugar addictive. Over time, the brain requires more sugar to achieve the same dopamine hit, creating a dependency cycle similar to that of addictive substances. This dependency doesn't just affect the brain; it can drive patterns of overeating and contribute to chronic health issues like obesity and diabetes.

Sugar isn't just toxic to our metabolic health; it also disrupts the delicate balance of our gut microbiome. Our digestive system is home to trillions of bacteria, many of which play essential roles in digestion, immunity, and even mood regulation. However, sugar creates an environment that favors the growth of harmful microbes, such as *Candida* and other sugar-dependent bacteria. These harmful microbes feed on sugar and can overpopulate, leading to dysbiosis—a bacterial imbalance that disrupts gut health.

Dysbiosis compromises the gut lining, weakens immune defenses, and disrupts the gut-brain axis, the communication channel between the brain and digestive system. This imbalance can negatively affect mental health, leading to symptoms like anxiety, fatigue, and mood swings, as well as physical symptoms, such as bloating and inflammation.

One of the most toxic effects of sugar is its role in promoting inflammation. When sugar enters the bloodstream in high amounts, it triggers the release of inflammatory cytokines, chemicals that can damage tissues and organs over time. Chronic inflammation has been linked to numerous serious health conditions, including heart disease, cancer, and autoimmune disorders. For individuals dealing with chronic health issues, reducing sugar intake is often a foundational step toward managing inflammation and improving overall health.

Furthermore, excess sugar consumption suppresses the immune system, making the body more vulnerable to infections. This is especially concerning during times of stress or illness, when the body needs a robust immune response. Studies show that even a moderate amount of sugar can weaken the immune system for several hours after consumption, impairing the body's ability to fight off pathogens.

THE GUT-BRAIN AXIS AND MENTAL HEALTH

The gut-brain axis is a two-way communication channel that links gut health with brain function. A healthy gut supports stable mood and mental clarity, but an imbalanced gut microbiome can contribute to anxiety, depression, and other mood disorders. Harmful bacteria that thrive on sugar disrupt this gut-brain communication by producing neurochemicals that interfere with mental well-being. When the gut bacteria are out of balance, they may produce less serotonin and dopamine—the neurotransmitters responsible for happiness and emotional stability—contributing to mental health challenges.

Minimizing sugar intake and prioritizing gut health are essential steps in protecting your body from sugar's toxic effects. Breaking free from sugar dependency not only improves digestion and immune strength but also enhances mental clarity, energy, and emotional resilience. In the next section we'll explore lifestyle changes that are foundational to a healthier, more balanced body, empowering you to live with greater vitality and reduced risk of sugar-related health issues.

Understanding Gut Health and Detoxification

Your gut is much more than a part of the digestive system—it's a key player in detoxification, immune health, and even weight management. When we talk about gut health, we're really referring to the health of the gut microbiome, the vast ecosystem of bacteria and other microorganisms that live in your digestive tract. A healthy, balanced gut microbiome is essential for breaking down food, absorbing nutrients, supporting immune function, and eliminating toxins. Unfortunately, imbalances in the gut, often caused by factors like poor diet, stress, or even parasites, can lead to weight gain, toxin buildup, and health issues. Let's dive into how gut health affects detox and weight loss, and explore some strategies for keeping your microbiome balanced.

The gut microbiome is made up of trillions of microorganisms, including bacteria, fungi, and viruses, that live in harmony in a healthy digestive tract. These "friendly" bacteria play a critical role in our overall health:

Breaking Down Food Gut bacteria help break down complex carbohydrates, fibers, and other substances that our bodies can't digest on their own. This process releases important nutrients and produces beneficial compounds like short-chain fatty acids, which support gut health and reduce inflammation.

Supporting Detoxification The gut helps process and eliminate waste products, including toxins. The liver breaks down many toxins and sends them to the intestines to be excreted. A healthy gut microbiome assists this process, helping prevent toxins from being reabsorbed into the body.

Regulating Metabolism and Weight Certain gut bacteria play a role in how efficiently we use and store energy. Studies have shown that people with a more diverse microbiome (a greater variety of bacterial species) tend to have healthier weights, while those with less diversity may be more prone to weight gain. Some gut bacteria are involved in hormone regulation, influencing hunger, satiety, and cravings. When the gut microbiome is balanced, these bacteria help regulate appetite and support a healthy metabolism, which can make weight loss easier.

A balanced, healthy gut microbiome is like a well-functioning filter—it helps the body get rid of what it doesn't need while absorbing what it does need. But when the gut microbiome becomes imbalanced, it can allow harmful substances to accumulate, which strains the body's detox pathways and may lead to weight gain and other health problems.

PARASITES AND MICROBIAL IMBALANCE

An imbalance in the gut microbiome, often referred to as *dysbiosis*, occurs when harmful bacteria outnumber the beneficial bacteria. This imbalance can lead to a number of issues that interfere with detoxification and weight management. In addition, the presence of parasites in the gut can further disrupt the microbiome and contribute to health problems.

Parasites Parasites are organisms that live off their host—in this case, the human body. Certain parasites can reside in the intestines, where they consume nutrients from the food we eat, depleting the body of essential nutrients. Parasites also produce waste products that can be toxic and inflammatory, adding to the body's toxin load. They may lead to digestive discomfort, cravings, and nutrient deficiencies, all of which can make it more challenging to lose weight and feel well.

Harmful Bacteria and Dysbiosis When there are too many harmful bacteria or not enough beneficial bacteria, the gut becomes a less effective detoxifier. Harmful bacteria can produce toxic byproducts, increase inflammation, and damage the lining of the gut. This damage can lead to a condition called *leaky gut*, where toxins and undigested food particles "leak" through the gut lining and enter the bloodstream. Leaky gut is linked to chronic inflammation, immune dysfunction, and weight gain.

Increased Cravings and Poor Metabolism An imbalanced microbiome can disrupt the production of certain hormones and neurotransmitters involved in appetite regulation, mood, and energy. For example, certain types of bacteria produce short-chain fatty acids that signal fullness, while others influence the production of serotonin, a neurotransmitter that affects mood and cravings. When harmful bacteria overpopulate the gut, these beneficial processes are disrupted, potentially leading to overeating, cravings for unhealthy foods, and a sluggish metabolism.

Overall, an imbalanced gut, whether due to parasites or harmful bacteria, can increase the body's toxin load, weaken immunity, and make weight loss more difficult.

Fortunately, there are several strategies to restore and support a healthy gut microbiome. By incorporating certain foods and supplements, you can promote the growth of beneficial bacteria, reduce harmful bacteria, and support your body's detoxification processes.

Probiotics Probiotics are live beneficial bacteria that can help restore balance in the gut microbiome. They're found in fermented foods and supplements and work by introducing helpful bacteria that can crowd out harmful bacteria. Regular consumption of probiotics can improve digestion, reduce inflammation, and support the immune system.

Include fermented foods in your diet, such as yogurt, kefir, sauerkraut, kimchi, miso, and kombucha. These foods contain various strains of beneficial bacteria that can help diversify the microbiome.

For those who need an extra boost or are dealing with specific gut issues, probiotic supplements can help. Look for high-quality supplements that contain a variety of bacterial strains, such as Lactobacillus and Bifidobacterium.

Prebiotics Prebiotics are types of fiber that feed beneficial gut bacteria, helping them grow and thrive. By nourishing the good bacteria, prebiotics indirectly reduce harmful bacteria in the gut, promoting a balanced microbiome.

Foods high in prebiotics include garlic, onions, leeks, asparagus, bananas, apples, oats, and chicory root. Adding these foods to your diet helps create an environment where beneficial bacteria can flourish.

Nutrient-Dense, Anti-Inflammatory Foods A diet rich in nutrient-dense foods helps reduce inflammation, support detoxification, and promote a healthy microbiome. Focus on whole, unprocessed foods that are high in fiber, vitamins, and antioxidants.

Vegetables and Fruits Leafy greens, berries, and cruciferous vegetables (like broccoli and cauliflower) are high in fiber and antioxidants, which help support gut health and overall detoxification.

Healthy Fats Omega-3 fatty acids, found in foods like salmon, chia seeds, and walnuts, have anti-inflammatory properties that benefit gut health.

Lean Proteins Proteins are essential for tissue repair and immune function. Aim to include high-quality proteins, such as chicken, fish, beans, and legumes, to support gut health without overloading the digestive system.

Avoiding Trigger Foods Some foods can promote inflammation and encourage the growth of harmful bacteria. Reducing or avoiding processed foods, refined sugars, artificial sweeteners, and excessive alcohol can significantly improve gut health. These substances feed harmful bacteria and disrupt the microbiome, making it harder to maintain a balanced gut.

Hydration Staying hydrated is essential for gut health and detoxification. Water helps move waste through the digestive system and aids in maintaining a healthy balance of bacteria in the gut.

Regular Cleanses or Anti-Parasitic Protocols Certain herbs, like wormwood, black walnut, and clove, have natural anti-parasitic properties and can help reduce parasitic load. Periodic cleansing can help maintain gut balance and support detoxification. When there's an imbalance in our gut microbiome, harmful microbes like *Candida* often overgrow, feeding on sugars and amplifying cravings. By understanding the root causes of this imbalance, we can start to restore harmony in the gut, reduce sugar dependency, and support overall wellness.

Two effective approaches for rebalancing the gut include antimicrobial herbal tinctures and fasting protocols. Together, these strategies combat harmful microbes in unique ways, paving the way for a healthier, more balanced microbiome.

ANTIMICROBIAL TINCTURES FOR GUT HEALTH

Several antimicrobial herbal tinctures are known to help eliminate harmful bacteria, fungi, and yeast in the gut, especially those that thrive on sugar. Here are some of the most effective options:

Oregano Oil Tincture Oregano oil is rich in carvacrol and thymol, two potent compounds with antimicrobial, antifungal, and antiviral properties. It's particularly effective against Candida yeast overgrowth, as well as harmful bacteria. Take a few drops diluted in water (follow dosing on the label, as it can be strong). Use in cycles (e.g., 2-3 weeks on, 1-2 weeks off) to avoid overuse.

Garlic Tincture Garlic contains allicin, which has powerful antibacterial, antifungal, and antiparasitic effects. It's effective against harmful gut bacteria and yeast like Candida while leaving beneficial bacteria relatively unharmed. Start with a small dose (usually around 10-15 drops) and gradually increase, as garlic can be strong. Take it with food to reduce any potential digestive discomfort.

Berberine (from Goldenseal, Barberry, or Oregon Grape) Berberine is an alkaloid found in plants like goldenseal, barberry, and Oregon grape. It has broad-spectrum antimicrobial effects, targeting bacteria, fungi, and parasites. Studies show it's effective against various gut pathogens and may help rebalance the gut microbiome. Berberine tinctures should be used in cycles (2-3 weeks on, 1 week off). Start with a low dose and monitor your body's response, as it can be potent.

Pau D'Arco Tincture Derived from the bark of a South American tree, Pau D'Arco is a powerful antifungal and antibacterial agent, effective against yeast infections and certain bacterial strains. Take 1-2 droppers of Pau D'Arco tincture in water, 2-3 times per day. It can be used consistently for 2-4 weeks, but it's advisable to take breaks after extended use.

Clove Tincture Clove contains eugenol, a compound with strong antifungal, antibacterial, and antioxidant properties. Clove is especially useful against fungi like Candida, making it a great option for sugar-related gut imbalances. Clove tinctures are very potent, so start with 5-10 drops in water, 1-2 times daily, and adjust based on tolerance.

Black Walnut Hull Tincture Black walnut is highly effective against parasites, bacteria, and fungi. It's often used in combination with other antimicrobials for detox protocols, as it can help eliminate sugar-dependent microbes and rebalance the gut. Take 1-2 droppers in water, usually 2-3 times daily. Black walnut is strong, so follow label recommendations and avoid prolonged use without breaks.

Thyme Tincture Thyme is another herb high in thymol, an antimicrobial compound that can help eliminate harmful bacteria and fungi in the gut. It's effective against certain antibiotic-resistant bacteria and can support gut health. Take 1 dropper in water, 1-2 times per day. Thyme can be combined with oregano or other herbs for a broader effect.

Grapefruit Seed Extract (GSE) GSE has strong antibacterial and antifungal effects. It's often used to target Candida and other sugar-loving microbes. GSE tinctures are typically very concentrated, so start with a low dose (e.g., 5-10 drops in water) and increase as needed. It can be cycled for best results.

TIPS FOR USING ANTIMICROBIAL TINCTURES SAFELY

Cycle the Use To prevent microbial resistance and reduce strain on the liver, alternate between 2-3 weeks on and 1-2 weeks off, or as recommended.

Start Slowly Begin with a low dose and gradually increase to gauge tolerance.

Support Detoxification As microbes die off, toxins may be released, potentially causing symptoms like fatigue or headaches (known as "die-off" symptoms). Drinking plenty of water, getting enough rest, and incorporating liver-supporting herbs like milk thistle can help.

Combine with Probiotics Since antimicrobial herbs can impact some beneficial bacteria, consider supplementing with a high-quality probiotic to maintain balance in your gut flora.

These tinctures, when used mindfully and in cycles, can help cleanse the gut of harmful, sugar-dependent microbes and support a more balanced and resilient gut microbiome.

STARVING HARMFUL BACTERIA AND SUPPORTING HEALING WITH FASTING

Fasting works by depriving harmful bacteria of their main fuel source—sugar—while shifting the body's energy metabolism from glucose to ketones. This metabolic switch creates an environment less hospitable to sugar-loving microbes and activates the body's natural detoxification processes, supporting microbial balance and gut health.

Ketosis and Microbial Balance During fasting, glucose levels drop, depriving harmful microbes of their primary fuel. The body then produces ketones, which not only provide an alternative energy source but also reduce inflammation. By favoring ketone-based energy, fasting promotes an internal environment where beneficial bacteria can thrive, tipping the scales toward a balanced microbiome.

Autophagy and Cellular Detox Fasting also initiates autophagy, a cellular "cleanup" process where old, damaged cells are broken down and recycled. In the gut, autophagy helps eliminate inflamed or damaged cells caused by microbial imbalance, creating a more favorable environment for beneficial bacteria to flourish.

TYPES OF FASTING FOR GUT HEALTH

Intermittent Fasting (16–24 Hours) For beginners, a 16- to 24-hour fast is manageable and helps initiate autophagy. This approach weakens harmful bacteria by reducing their access to glucose and provides beneficial bacteria with a chance to repopulate.

Extended Fasting (48–72 Hours) More experienced fasters can benefit from a 48- to 72-hour fast, which enhances autophagy and growth hormone production for deeper cellular repair. Extended fasting is particularly effective in reducing bacterial overgrowth and supporting the immune system.

Water Fasting A water-only fast is the most intensive approach for addressing microbial overgrowth, as it eliminates all sources of nutrients for harmful bacteria. Due to its intensity, water fasting should be supervised by a healthcare provider.

During fasting, staying hydrated is essential. Herbal teas, like chamomile or ginger, provide additional anti-inflammatory support, while diluted apple cider vinegar can add mild antimicrobial benefits. After a fast, reintroduce food slowly, focusing on prebiotic-rich vegetables and probiotic foods to establish and maintain a balanced microbiome.

By combining antimicrobial herbal tinctures with fasting, you create a powerful one-two punch against harmful gut microbes. Herbal tinctures work directly on reducing harmful bacteria and fungi, while fasting limits their fuel source and activates the body's natural repair processes. Taking these steps not only supports a balanced microbiome but also builds resilience in the body, fostering better digestion, immunity, and mental clarity.

Apple cider vinegar (ACV) can have a similar, albeit milder, effect in helping reduce the overgrowth of harmful bacteria, fungi, and yeast in the gut. While ACV may not be as potent as some herbal tinctures specifically known for their antimicrobial properties, it still offers several benefits that support gut health and reduce sugar-loving microbes. Here's how ACV can help:

Antimicrobial Properties ACV contains acetic acid, which has natural antimicrobial effects that can help inhibit the growth of harmful bacteria and fungi. Studies show that acetic acid can suppress pathogens like *E. coli*, *Candida albicans*, and *Staphylococcus aureus*. This antimicrobial effect may help to reduce sugar-dependent microbes, especially when used regularly in small amounts as part of a balanced diet.

Promotes Healthy Gut pH The acetic acid in ACV can help lower the pH of the gut slightly, creating an environment that is less favorable for pathogenic bacteria and yeast to thrive. Many harmful microbes prefer a more alkaline environment, so a slightly acidic pH can help keep them in check.

Supports Digestion and Reduces Sugar Cravings ACV has been shown to help regulate blood sugar levels by slowing down the rate at which sugars and other carbohydrates are digested. Improved digestion and blood sugar regulation can support overall gut health and reduce the likelihood of microbial imbalances.

Encourages Healthy Bacteria Growth Raw, unfiltered ACV contains beneficial bacteria (probiotics) from the "mother," a collection of proteins, enzymes, and friendly bacteria. Though not as concentrated as a probiotic supplement, these beneficial bacteria can support a healthier gut microbiome and crowd out harmful microbes over time.

Anti-Inflammatory and Detoxifying Effects ACV has mild anti-inflammatory properties, which can help reduce inflammation in the gut caused by microbial imbalances or "die-off" reactions (when harmful bacteria or yeast die and release toxins). ACV can also support liver function and aid the body's natural detoxification processes, helping to eliminate microbial byproducts and toxins more effectively.

If you're not used to taking ACV, start with 1 teaspoon in a glass of water and gradually work up to 1–2 tablespoons to avoid potential digestive discomfort. Always dilute ACV in water to protect your teeth and esophagus from the acidity. While ACV is beneficial, combining it with other antimicrobial herbs (like oregano, garlic, or berberine) may provide more targeted effects for tackling sugar-loving microbes.

Apple cider vinegar can be a great addition to a gut-healing and sugar-reducing protocol. Although it's not as potent as certain antimicrobial tinctures, it offers a range of benefits for balancing gut health, supporting digestion, and reducing sugar cravings. Regular use of ACV, combined with other antimicrobial herbs, a balanced diet, and probiotics, can make a meaningful impact on managing sugar-loving microbes and improving gut resilience.

By supporting your gut health through these strategies, you'll create a balanced, thriving microbiome that can aid in detoxification, improve metabolism, and help you achieve and maintain a healthy weight. A healthy gut isn't just about digestion—it's a foundation for your overall wellness and vitality.

Nutrition for Detox and Weight Loss

Nutrition is one of the most powerful tools for supporting your body's natural detoxification processes and achieving sustainable weight loss. By making strategic dietary choices, you can encourage your body to eliminate toxins, regulate metabolism, and maintain energy balance.

Carbohydrates, especially refined carbs like sugar and white flour, cause spikes in blood sugar, which leads to increased insulin production. Insulin is a hormone that regulates blood sugar levels but also encourages fat storage. When carb intake is reduced, insulin levels decrease, making it easier for the body to access and burn stored fat for energy.

Low-carb diets focus on reducing carbohydrate intake, especially refined carbs and sugars, and instead prioritize protein and healthy fats. This dietary approach can be highly effective for weight loss and detoxification due to its unique effects on metabolism and toxin storage.

With fewer carbs, the body is forced to use fat as its primary fuel source, a state known as ketosis. When the body is in ketosis, it not only burns stored fat but also avoids the blood sugar highs and lows that can lead to cravings and overeating. This fat-burning mode is also beneficial for detox, as toxins are often stored in fat cells. By burning fat, the body releases these toxins, which can then be processed and eliminated.

A low-carb diet helps the body shed excess weight by targeting fat stores and stabilizing blood sugar, and it reduces the toxic load by helping release stored toxins. Opting for whole, unprocessed foods like lean proteins, healthy fats, and non-starchy vegetables can further support these benefits, making the body feel lighter and more energized.

Fasting and Low-Calorie Diets for Detoxification

Caloric restriction and intermittent fasting are powerful tools for enhancing detoxification and supporting weight loss. These approaches involve either reducing your overall caloric intake or limiting the hours during which you eat. Here's how they benefit your body:

Autophagy: The Cellular "Clean-Up"

When you fast or reduce calories, your body initiates a process called autophagy, where cells break down and remove damaged components. This cellular "clean-up" helps clear out toxins, reduce oxidative stress, and renew cellular function. By giving the digestive system a break, fasting allows the body to focus on eliminating stored toxins and enhancing cellular health.

Weight Loss and Fat-Stored Toxins

Fasting and caloric restriction also support weight loss by improving insulin sensitivity and encouraging the body to use stored fat for energy (a state called ketosis). This process not only promotes a leaner body composition but also helps eliminate fat-stored toxins, making it an effective method for those aiming to lose weight and detox simultaneously.

Intermittent Fasting (IF) Intermittent fasting involves alternating between periods of eating and fasting. Popular patterns include 16:8 (16 hours of fasting, with an 8-hour eating window) or 18:6. During fasting periods, the body shifts its focus from digestion to cellular repair and maintenance. Without a constant influx of food, the body uses stored energy (fat) and activates detoxification processes at the cellular level.

Caloric Restriction Reducing your caloric intake, either daily or on certain days of the week, is known to support longevity and metabolic health. By lowering calorie intake, you reduce oxidative stress and inflammation, giving cells a break from constant energy processing. This rest period allows the body to prioritize cellular repair and rejuvenation.

Time-Restricted Eating This approach limits food intake to specific hours of the day, such as eating only between 10 a.m. and 6 p.m. Aligning with natural circadian rhythms, time-restricted eating promotes better digestion and metabolism. It also supports metabolic health by preventing overeating and creating a daily fasting window, during which the body can focus on internal maintenance.

By regularly engaging autophagy through these dietary practices, you enable your body to "take out the trash" at a cellular level, supporting detoxification and long-term wellness. Triggering autophagy consistently helps the body maintain a cleaner, more efficient cellular environment, which promotes sustained energy, resilience, and healthier aging.

Below is a picture of a domestic dog that was placed on a low-calorie, all-natural keto diet for 18 months and experienced a tremendous decrease in the size of a tumor that was growing on its lip:

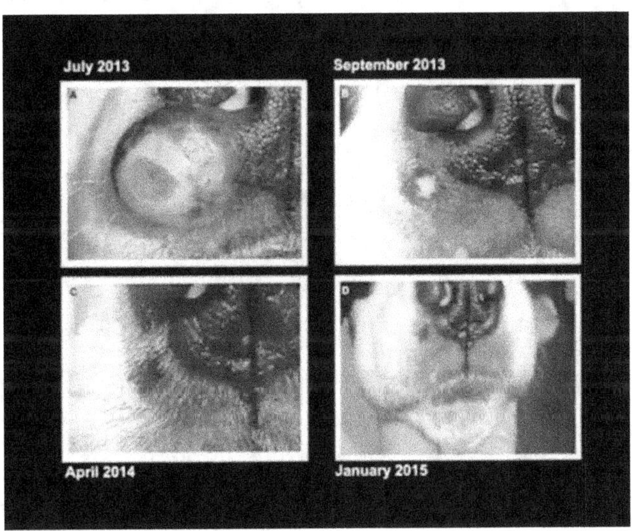

DETOX-FRIENDLY FOOD

Incorporating specific foods into your diet can further support the detox process and weight loss. These foods are rich in antioxidants, fiber, vitamins, and minerals that nourish the body and aid in toxin elimination. Here are some of the best detox-friendly foods:

Leafy Greens Spinach, kale, arugula, and other leafy greens are high in chlorophyll, which helps to remove heavy metals and other toxins from the body. They are also alkaline, which supports a balanced pH and reduces inflammation.

Fiber-Rich Vegetables Fiber binds to toxins in the digestive tract, helping the body eliminate them through stool. Fiber also supports a healthy gut microbiome, which is essential for overall detox. Good sources of fiber-rich vegetables include broccoli, cauliflower, Brussels sprouts, carrots, and beets.

Antioxidant-Rich Fruits Blueberries, strawberries, and raspberries are packed with antioxidants, which help protect cells from oxidative damage and support the body's detoxification pathways. Antioxidants neutralize free radicals, which are harmful molecules that can damage cells and contribute to aging and disease.

Garlic and Onions These foods contain sulfur compounds that support liver function and help the liver process and eliminate toxins. Garlic also has antibacterial properties that can support gut health and reduce harmful bacteria.

Ginger and Turmeric Both ginger and turmeric have anti-inflammatory and antioxidant properties. Ginger aids digestion, while turmeric supports liver health and promotes healthy inflammatory responses, making them both valuable for detox and weight loss.

Cruciferous Vegetables Vegetables like broccoli, cabbage, cauliflower and kale contain compounds that promote the production of enzymes that help the liver detoxify the body. They are also high in fiber, which aids in waste elimination.

Green Tea Green tea is high in catechins, a type of antioxidant that enhances liver function. It also has mild diuretic properties that help flush out toxins through urine.

Citrus Fruits Lemons, limes, and oranges are high in vitamin C, which supports the immune system and enhances liver function. Adding lemon to water can also stimulate digestion and support hydration, which is essential for detox.

By including these foods in your diet, you're supporting the body's detox systems—particularly the liver, kidneys, and lymphatic system—and helping create an environment where weight loss and toxin elimination are possible. These foods provide the body with the nutrients needed to flush out waste, reduce inflammation, and maintain a healthy weight.

Combining a low-carb approach with caloric restriction, intermittent fasting, and a diet rich in detox-friendly foods creates a powerful strategy for detoxification and weight loss. By adopting these practices, you give your body the tools it needs to break down fat, eliminate toxins, and reset its natural processes. Detox-friendly foods add essential nutrients that protect and support key detox organs, while fasting and caloric restriction stimulate autophagy, helping your cells stay healthy, clean, and energized.

Remember, detoxing is not about quick fixes but rather about making lasting changes that support your body's health and resilience over time. By nourishing your body and practicing mindful eating, you create a foundation for sustainable weight loss and overall wellness.

Nourishing Recipes

Eliminating processed foods and refined sugars is a powerful step toward healing and can make a significant difference in your journey to wellness. By choosing whole, nutrient-dense foods, you'll support your body's natural detox processes, boost energy levels, and promote mental clarity.

These wholesome recipes are crafted with nutrient-rich ingredients like leafy greens, root vegetables, and healing spices. Each ingredient has been carefully selected to support the lymphatic system, aiding in the gentle removal of toxins and promoting overall well-being. The recipes are designed not only to nourish but to comfort and energize you with every bite.

Each recipe is simple to prepare and crafted to help your body function at its best by enhancing your natural detox processes. As you enjoy these meals, you're not only nourishing your body but also giving your lymphatic system the support it needs to help clear toxins effectively. Whether you're in the mood for a light, refreshing soup or a hearty, restorative stew, this collection has something to meet your needs and cravings.

Tonics and Juices

Detox Water Tonic Combine sliced lemon and cucumber with a handful of mint leaves and filtered water. Optionally, add a 1-inch piece of peeled and sliced ginger. Store in a pitcher and let infuse in the refrigerator for at least 2 hours before serving.

Turmeric & Coconut Tonic 1 tsp turmeric powder, 1-inch piece of ginger, grated. Pinch of cayenne pepper, 1 C. coconut water. Combine all the ingredients in a pitcher and let infuse in the refrigerator for at least 2 hours before serving.

Lemon Water with Cayenne Pepper Tonic Juice from 1 lemon, 4 C. filtered water. Pinch of cayenne pepper. Combine all the ingredients in a pitcher and drink first thing in the morning, on an empty stomach.

Detox Green Juice Use any desired combination of kale and/or spinach, celery, cucumber, and apple, lemon and ginger. Add to a juicer machine and serve immediately over ice or store for not more than 24 hours in the refrigerator.

Bowls & Smoothies

Green Smoothie Kale, cucumber, spinach, juice from 1 lemon or lime, 1-inch piece of ginger, peeled and sliced & 1 C. water, coconut water, regular filtered water or ice. Blend all the ingredients together until smooth, serve immediately.

Berry Smoothie Bowl Blend frozen chunks of banana, mixed berries, almond milk, and a scoop of protein powder until smooth. Pour into a bowl and top with your choice of granola, sliced almonds, sunflower seeds, walnuts and additional berries for a refreshing and energizing meal.

Anti-Inflammatory Smoothie 1 C. mixed berries, 1 T. flaxseed oil or CoQ10 oil, 1 tsp. turmeric powder, 1 C. coconut milk. Blend all the ingredients together until smooth, serve immediately.

Almond Butter Banana Smoothie Bowl Blend almond butter, frozen chunks of banana, almond or coconut milk, and chia seeds until smooth. Add more milk if needed for desired consistency.

Green Detox Smoothie Bowl 1 C. spinach, 1 banana, cut into chunks and frozen, 1/2 avocado 1 T. chia seeds, 1 C. coconut water, filtered water, or ice. Blend all ingredients until smooth and serve. Optionally, add nuts and seeds on top.

Tropical Sweet Green Smoothie Blend your choice of spinach, kale, cucumber, frozen chunks of banana, pineapple chunks, pineapple juice, orange juice, coconut milk, and almond milk together until smooth and serve immediately.

Acai Bowl with Pumpkin Seeds Blend your choice of acai puree, fresh or frozen berries, frozen chunks of banana, with almond, coconut milk, yogurt, ice or filtered water until smooth. Pour into a bowl and top with fresh or roasted and salted pumpkin seeds.

Cucumber and Mint Smoothie Blend your choice of cucumber, mint, pineapple fruit or juice, and coconut or filtered water or ice together until smooth and serve immediately.

Breakfast

Quinoa Porridge with Coconut Milk Cook quinoa according to package instructions, using coconut milk instead of water. Stir in cinnamon, nutmeg, and raisins before serving.

Turmeric Ginger Oatmeal Cook oats with powdered turmeric and ginger, add almond milk. Sweeten with your choice of sweetener and serve hot.

Breakfast Casserole Eggs, ground turkey, bell peppers, onions, spinach, coconut oil. Preheat oven to 375°F. In a skillet, cook ground turkey until browned. Add in diced vegetables and cook until softened. In a mixing bowl, whisk eggs and pour over the turkey and vegetable mixture. Bake in the oven for 25-30 minutes or until eggs are cooked through.

Cauliflower Breakfast Hash Cauliflower, bacon, onions, bell peppers, garlic, eggs. In a skillet, cook bacon until crispy. Add in diced cauliflower, onions, bell peppers, and garlic. Cook until vegetables are tender. Push vegetables to the side of the skillet and crack eggs into the center. Cook until eggs are done to your liking.

Sweet Potato Breakfast Bowl Sweet potato, avocado, bacon, eggs, spinach. Cook bacon in a skillet until crispy. In the same skillet, cook diced sweet potato until soft. Remove sweet potato and cook eggs to your liking. Assemble the breakfast bowl with cooked sweet potato, avocado slices, eggs, bacon, and spinach.

Bacon and Egg Bites Eggs, bacon, spinach, cherry tomatoes. Preheat oven to 350℉. Grease a muffin tin with coconut oil. Line each cup with cooked bacon strips. Crack an egg into each cup. Bake in the oven for 15-20 minutes or until eggs are set.

Breakfast Burrito Eggs, bell peppers, onions, avocado, bacon, coconut oil. In a skillet, cook diced bell peppers and onions until softened. Add in beaten eggs and scramble until cooked. Fill a coconut flour tortilla with the egg mixture, sliced avocado, and cooked bacon. Roll up and enjoy.

Smoked Salmon and Avocado Toast Smoked salmon, avocado, coconut flour toast, lemon juice. Toast coconut flour bread slices until crispy. Mash avocado and spread on each toast. Top with slices of smoked salmon and a squeeze of lemon juice.

Zucchini Noodle Egg Scramble Zucchini noodles, eggs, cherry tomatoes, spinach, coconut oil. In a skillet, sauté zucchini noodles until slightly softened. Add in beaten eggs, cherry tomatoes, and spinach. Cook until eggs are set and vegetables are cooked through.

Sausage & Veggie Breakfast Skillet Sausage, bell peppers, onions, mushrooms, eggs. In a skillet, cook sausage until browned. Add in diced vegetables and cook until softened. Crack eggs into the skillet and cook until set. Serve hot.

Avocado & Micro Greens Toast Whole grain bread, avocado, microgreens, lemon juice, sea salt. Toast bread and mash avocado on top. Squeeze lemon juice over the avocado, sprinkle with sea salt, and top with microgreens.

Broccoli & Spinach Frittata Eggs, broccoli, spinach, feta cheese, olive oil. Beat eggs and mix with broccoli, spinach, and feta cheese. Pour into a greased baking dish and bake at 375°F for 25-30 minutes, or until set. Serve hot.

Salads

Spinach and Mango Salad Combine spinach, mango, red onion, pumpkin seeds, lemon juice, olive oil, sea salt

Avocado and Grapefruit Salad Combine 1 avocado, diced, 1 grapefruit, segmented, mixed greens & lemon vinaigrette (made with lemon juice, olive oil, salt, and pepper)

Detoxifying Green Salad Combine mixed greens, cucumber, avocado, cilantro, lemon juice, olive oil, sea salt. Top with toasted seeds like pumpkin and sunflower.

Beet and Chickpea Salad Combine 1 can chickpeas, rinsed and drained, 2 medium beets, roasted and chopped 1/4 C. chopped fresh mint, 1/4 cup crumbled feta cheese, 2 T. olive oil, juice of 1 lemon, and salt and pepper to taste.

Avocado and Kale Salad Combine 1 bunch kale, stems removed and chopped, 1 avocado, diced, 1/4 C. pumpkin seeds, 2 T. olive oil, juice of 1 lemon, salt and pepper to taste.

Cucumber and Fennel Salad Combine 1 cucumber, thinly sliced, 1 fennel bulb, thinly sliced, 1/4 C. chopped fresh dill, 2 T. olive oil, juice of 1 lemon, salt and pepper to taste.

Vinaigrette Salad Dressing Combine apple cider vinegar, olive oil, and a touch of maple syrup.

Honey Dijon Vinaigrette Salad Dressing Combine apple cider vinegar, Dijon mustard, honey, olive oil, sea salt

Turmeric Carrot Ginger Soup

- 6 carrots, chopped
- 1 onion, chopped
- 3 cloves of garlic, minced
- 1 inch piece of ginger, grated
- 1 tsp of turmeric
- 4 cups of vegetable broth
- Salt and pepper to taste

In a large pot, sauté the onion and garlic until fragrant. Add in the chopped carrots and ginger, and cook for a few minutes. Stir in the turmeric and vegetable broth. Bring the mixture to a boil, then reduce the heat and let it simmer for about 20 minutes. Use an immersion blender to blend the soup until smooth. Season with salt and pepper before serving.

Lentil Curry Cook lentils with a blend of curry spices like turmeric, cumin, and coriander, then add coconut milk & roasted cauliflower.

Sweet Potato and Butternut Squash Soup

- 1 sweet potato, peeled and chopped
- 1 butternut squash, peeled and chopped
- 1 onion, chopped
- 3 cloves of garlic, minced
- 4 cups of vegetable broth
- Salt and pepper to taste

In a large pot, sauté the onion and garlic until softened. Add in the chopped sweet potato, butternut squash, and vegetable broth. Bring the mixture to a boil, then reduce the heat and let it simmer for about 30 minutes. Use an immersion blender to blend the soup until smooth. Season with salt and pepper before serving.

Turmeric Coconut Milk Broth This warming, nourishing dish with anti-inflammatory benefits from the turmeric is balanced by the rich creaminess of coconut milk. Enjoyed on its own or as a base for soups, noodles, or curries.

- 1 T. coconut oil (or olive oil)
- 1 small onion, finely chopped
- 3 cloves garlic, minced
- 1-inch piece of fresh ginger, peeled and grated
- 1 T. turmeric powder (or 1-inch fresh turmeric, grated)
- 1 tsp ground cumin
- 1 tsp ground coriander
- ½ tsp ground black pepper (increases the bioavailability of turmeric)
- 1 can (400 ml) full-fat coconut milk
- 3 C. vegetable or chicken broth
- 1 T. soy sauce or tamari (optional for saltiness)
- 1 T. lime juice (or lemon juice)
- Salt to taste

Sauté the Aromatics In a medium saucepan or pot, heat the coconut oil over medium heat. Add the chopped onion and sauté for about 3-4 minutes until soft and translucent. Add the minced garlic, grated ginger, and grated fresh turmeric (or turmeric powder). Sauté for another 1-2 minutes until fragrant, but be careful not to let the garlic burn. **Add Spices:** Stir in the ground cumin, ground coriander, and black pepper. Let the spices toast for 30 seconds to release their aromas. **Pour in Coconut Milk & Broth:** Add the coconut milk and vegetable (or chicken) broth to the pot. Stir well to combine, making sure the spices are fully incorporated. **Simmer the Broth:** Bring the mixture to a gentle simmer. Let it cook for 10-15 minutes, allowing the flavors to meld together. Stir occasionally to prevent sticking at the bottom. **Season:** Stir in the soy sauce or tamari (if using), lime juice, and salt to taste. Adjust the seasoning to your preference, adding more lime juice for acidity or salt for flavor. **Serve:** Ladle the turmeric coconut broth into bowls. This broth pairs well with noodles or can be enjoyed as a light soup on its own.

Side Dishes

Roasted Brussels Sprouts Cut Brussels sprouts in half, toss with olive oil, balsamic vinegar, and a sprinkle of sea salt. Roast in the oven until caramelized and crispy for a delicious and healthy side dish.

Lemon Turmeric Roasted Cauliflower Combine 1 head cauliflower, cut into florets, juice from 1 lemon, 1 tsp. Turmeric, 1 T. olive oil, with salt and pepper to taste. Preheat the oven or air fryer to 360°F. Cook for 15-20 minutes, or until the cauliflower is golden brown.

Detoxifying Broccoli and Kale Stir-Fry Combine broccoli, kale, bell peppers, garlic, ginger, tamari sauce, sesame oil, rice vinegar

Vegetable Stir-Fry Saute a mixture of colorful vegetables such as broccoli, bell peppers, snap peas, and mushrooms in a little coconut oil. Season with garlic, ginger, and tamari sauce.

Zucchini Noodles with Pesto Spiralize zucchini into noodles and toss with homemade pesto made from fresh basil, garlic, pine nuts, and olive oil. Top with cherry tomatoes and a sprinkle of nutritional yeast.

Salmon with Roasted Vegetables Salmon filets, asparagus, trimmed, sliced red and yellow bell pepper and sliced zucchini, 2 T. olive oil, 1 tsp dried dill, salt and pepper to taste. Preheat the air fryer to 360°F. Place the salmon filet in the air fryer basket, layer veggies on top. Cook for 15-20 minutes, or until the salmon is cooked through.

Lemon Garlic Baked Fish Salmon or cod filet, 1 lemon, 2 cloves garlic, minced, salt and pepper to taste. Preheat the air fryer to 360°F. Place the salmon filet in the air fryer basket. Squeeze the juice of the lemon over the salmon. Sprinkle minced garlic, salt, and pepper over the salmon. Cook for 15-20 minutes, or until the salmon is cooked through.

Herb Roasted Chicken Breast 2 chicken breasts, 1 T. olive oil, 1 tsp. dried thyme, 1 tsp. dried rosemary, salt and pepper to taste. Preheat the air fryer to 360°F. Rub the chicken breasts with olive oil. Season with thyme, rosemary, salt, and pepper. Place the chicken breasts in the air fryer basket. Cook for 20-25 minutes, or until the chicken is cooked through.

Quinoa Stuffed Bell Peppers 4 bell peppers, 1 C. cooked quinoa, 1 can black beans (rinsed and drained), 1 C. pico de gallo or salsa, 1 tsp. cumin, salt and pepper to taste. Cut the tops off the bell peppers and remove the seeds. In a bowl, mix quinoa, black beans, salsa, cumin, salt, and pepper. Stuff each bell pepper with the quinoa mixture. Place the stuffed bell peppers in the air fryer basket. Cook for 15-20 minutes, or until the peppers are tender.

Spinach and Mushroom Stuffed Chicken Breasts 1-2 chicken breasts, chopped spinach, sliced mushrooms, olive oil, salt and pepper to taste. Preheat the air fryer to 360°F. In a skillet, sauté spinach and mushrooms in olive oil until cooked. Cut a pocket in each chicken breast and stuff with the spinach and mushroom mixture. Place the stuffed chicken breasts in the air fryer basket. Cook for 25-30 minutes, or until the chicken is cooked through.

Barria Cauliflower Rice Bowls Soak any combination of 12 dried ancho and/or guajillo chiles (available in specialty stores or on Amazon) in water for 20 minutes, then remove the chile stems and shake out most of the seeds. Heat one can of chicken broth in a saucepan and add the rehydrated chiles to the pan, remove from heat and allow to soak for 20 more minutes. Add the chicken broth and chiles to a blender or food processor and add 2 T. each apple cider vinegar, salt, and honey, plus 1 T. each black pepper, cumin, oregano, and 1/2 T. each ginger and cinnamon. Add 6-8 crushed cloves of garlic, and 3-4 bay leaves. Blend on low for at least 1 minute. Put 4 lbs. of chicken breast or pot roast into a slow cooker. Add 1-2 large diced onions and 2-10 oz. cans of tomatoes. Pour the chile mixture from the blender over the top of the mixture into the slow cooker and cook on low setting for 6 to 8 hours. Shred with two forks inside the slow cooker and serve in bowls over cauliflower rice (frozen or homemade) with optional desired toppings (cilantro, avocado, sweet pickled red onions, lime, diced onions, cheese).

Thai Style Peanut Chicken Combine 3 lbs of dark or light meat chicken, one can of pure coconut milk, one cup of all-natural peanut butter (preferably chunky), 6-8 cloves of chopped garlic, 2 T. each honey, soy sauce, and rice wine vinegar or apple cider vinegar, juice from 1-2 limes, and 1 tsp. crushed red chili flakes or garlic chili paste. Cook in a slow cooker on low for 6 hours, stirring occasionally. Serve in lettuce cups with or without optional cauliflower rice or cooked rice noodles.

Cincinnati Chili Combine 1 lb. each ground turkey and/or 80/20 ground beef (2 lbs. total) browned and drained, with 1-2 large white onions, diced, and 3-6 cloves of freshly minced garlic, one can of tomato paste (5 oz.), 4 C. water, 1 T. each apple cider vinegar, Worcestershire sauce (optional, to taste), ½ T. salt, and 1 tsp. each ground cinnamon, ground cumin, and black pepper,

½ tsp. allspice, ¼ tsp. each cayenne pepper and paprika, 1-2 squares of unsweetened chocolate bar, and 8-12 finely chopped dried cloves. Cook in a slow cooker on low for 6 hours, stirring occasionally. Serve alone, or over cooked elbow macaroni or spaghetti noodles, with your choice of toppings: Finely shredded extra sharp cheddar, oyster crackers, crushed saltine crackers, cooked kidney beans and/or chopped onion.

Chicken Coconut Red Curry Soup In a Dutch oven or other heavy pot, heat the 1-2 T. olive oil over medium heat. Add 1 large onion, 2 large carrots, 1 of each red, yellow and green bell peppers, all chopped into large 1-inch pieces. Add a pinch of salt. Continue to cook, stirring occasionally, until the onion is translucent, about 5 to 8 minutes. Add 3-6 cloves of fresh garlic and ½-1 inch of peeled and shredded fresh ginger. Stir for roughly 30 seconds, not longer or the garlic will start to burn. Pour into a slow cooker with 4 C. of chicken stock and 1 can of fresh coconut milk, and 1 T. fish sauce (optional). Add in 1 T. red curry paste (sold in a tiny jar, refrigerated when not in use). Increase the heat to medium-high, and bring to a boil. In a second pan, brown 1-inch pieces of chicken breast until seared on all sides, combine chicken pieces with coconut mixture. Cook partially covered on medium heat until the soup has thickened slightly and the flavors come together, about 2 hours. Serve in

soup bowls, optionally over cooked frozen or homemade
cauliflower rice.

Desserts

These delicious, naturally sweetened, no-sugar dessert options satisfy a sweet tooth without refined sugar.

Chia Seed Pudding Chia seeds are rich in fiber and omega-3s, and this pudding has a creamy, satisfying texture that feels indulgent without added sugar. Mix 3 tablespoons of chia seeds with 1 cup of almond or coconut milk. Add 1/2 teaspoon of vanilla extract and a dash of cinnamon. Let it sit in the refrigerator for at least 2 hours or overnight. Top with fresh berries, nuts, or coconut.

Banana Nice Cream Blend frozen banana slices with a dash of vanilla (optional) until smooth. For a chocolate flavor, add a tablespoon of unsweetened cocoa powder, or mix in frozen berries for a fruity twist.

Coconut Bliss Balls Mix 1 cup of shredded coconut with 1/2 cup almond flour, 2 tablespoons of coconut oil, and a few drops of vanilla extract. Add stevia or monk fruit sweetener to taste. Roll into balls and refrigerate for 30 minutes.

Avocado Chocolate Mousse Blend 1 ripe avocado, 2 T. unsweetened cocoa powder, 1/4 cup almond milk, and a pinch of sweetener of your choice. Chill for 30 minutes before serving

Baked Cinnamon Apples Preheat the oven to 350°F (175°C). Slice apples and arrange them on a baking sheet (Granny Smith, Honeycrisp or Pink Lady work best due to their natural tartness). Sprinkle with cinnamon and nutmeg. Bake for 15-20 minutes until soft.

Coconut Yogurt Parfait Layer unsweetened coconut yogurt with fresh berries, a sprinkle of chia seeds, and your favorite nuts or seeds.

Baked Pears with Walnuts and Cinnamon Halve pears and scoop out a small section of the core. Fill each pear half with a sprinkle of cinnamon, a spoonful of chopped walnuts, and drizzle with almond butter. Bake at 350°F (175°C) for 15-20 minutes.

Pumpkin Spice Energy Bites Combine 1 C. of almond flour, 1/4 cup pumpkin puree, and spices. Sweeten to taste with stevia or monk fruit. Roll into bite-sized balls and refrigerate.

Cinnamon Apple Chips Thinly slice apples and sprinkle with cinnamon. Bake at 200°F (93°C) for 2-3 hours until crisp

Berry Chia Pudding Mix 1/4 C. chia seeds with 1 C. unsweetened almond milk. Add mashed berries and let sit overnight. Top with fresh berries before serving

Creamy Banana Chia Pudding In a blender, combine the 1 ripe banana, 1 C. unsweetened almond milk, ½ tsp. vanilla extract, and a pinch of cinnamon. Blend until smooth. Add 3 T. chia seeds and stir well. Pour into a jar and refrigerate for at least 4 hours or overnight. Serve chilled, topped with fresh berries or nuts if desired.

Almond Butter Energy Bites In a large bowl, combine 1 C. rolled oats, ½ cup almond butter (or any nut butter), ¼ cup honey or maple syrup, ¼ cup dark chocolate chips (85% cocoa or higher), and 1 tsp. vanilla extract until mixed thoroughly. Roll mixture into small balls. Place on a plate lined with parchment paper and refrigerate for at least 30 minutes to firm up.

Hydration and Clean Water

Hydration is essential for life, and water plays a critical role in nearly every bodily function—from digestion to circulation, temperature regulation, and, importantly, detoxification. Without adequate water intake, our detox systems, including the kidneys and lymphatic system, cannot function optimally. In addition, the quality of the water we drink matters just as much as the quantity. Contaminants in tap and bottled water can introduce toxins into the body, potentially straining detox pathways rather than supporting them. In this section, we'll explore why clean water is vital for detoxification, the risks of common water contaminants, and safer alternatives for reducing toxin exposure.

Pure, clean water is essential for detoxification. It serves as a medium for transporting nutrients, waste products, and other substances throughout the body, playing a key role in flushing out toxins. Here's how hydration supports the detox systems in the body:

Kidney Health The kidneys are the body's main filtration organs. They process about 200 quarts of blood each day, removing waste products, excess salts, and toxins, which are then excreted in urine. Without enough water, the kidneys struggle to perform this filtration process efficiently. When you're dehydrated, your body produces less urine, making it harder for the kidneys to flush out waste, which can lead to a buildup of toxins in the body. Over time, inadequate hydration can contribute to kidney stones, urinary tract infections, and even chronic kidney disease.

Lymphatic System Support The lymphatic system is responsible for clearing toxins and waste from tissues, supporting immune function, and balancing bodily fluids. However, unlike the circulatory system, the lymphatic system doesn't have a central pump (like the heart) to keep lymph fluid moving. Hydration is crucial because it helps keep lymph fluid thin and flowing smoothly, which allows it to move more freely and efficiently through lymph vessels. When we're dehydrated, lymph fluid can become sluggish or stagnant, leading to a buildup of toxins, swelling, and reduced immune response.

Digestive System Function Water is also vital for digestion and elimination. It helps break down food, absorb nutrients, and transport waste out of the body through bowel movements. Inadequate hydration can lead to constipation, slowing down the body's natural waste removal process and allowing toxins to linger in the digestive tract.

In short, drinking enough clean water each day is one of the most straightforward ways to support your body's natural detox pathways, ensuring that waste products are efficiently processed and excreted.

While drinking plenty of water is essential, the quality of the water is equally important. Many types of tap and bottled water contain contaminants that can introduce harmful substances into the body. These contaminants place additional strain on the detox systems, particularly the liver and kidneys, which are forced to work harder to filter out these unwanted substances.

Here are some common contaminants found in tap and bottled water:

Chlorine Chlorine is commonly added to tap water to kill bacteria and prevent contamination. While it's effective as a disinfectant, chlorine can react with other compounds in water to form harmful byproducts known as trihalomethanes (THMs). These compounds are associated with an increased risk of cancer and may contribute to liver and kidney strain.

Fluoride Fluoride is often added to municipal water supplies to prevent tooth decay. However, excessive fluoride can have negative effects, particularly on the thyroid gland, which plays a key role in metabolism. High fluoride intake is also linked to weakened bones and dental fluorosis.

Lead Lead can leach into tap water from old pipes and plumbing systems, especially in older buildings. Lead exposure is toxic and can cause serious health issues, including neurological damage, kidney strain, and high blood pressure. The body cannot easily eliminate lead, which means it tends to accumulate over time, creating a heavy toxic burden.

Mercury and Arsenic These metals can contaminate water sources through industrial runoff, mining, and other environmental pollutants. Mercury exposure is associated with neurological and kidney damage, while arsenic is a known carcinogen that affects multiple organs and increases cancer risk.

Microplastics Microplastics are tiny particles of plastic that enter water supplies through plastic waste, industrial runoff, and even degradation of bottled water containers. These particles are difficult for the body to break down and eliminate, and their long-term health effects are still being studied. Microplastics are believed to disrupt hormones and may contribute to inflammation, impacting metabolic health and detoxification pathways. Research has found that a significant portion of bottled water also contains microplastics due to the packaging and production processes.

Pharmaceutical Residues Traces of pharmaceuticals, such as antibiotics, hormones, and painkillers, are sometimes found in tap water due to improper disposal of medications and incomplete filtration at water treatment plants. These compounds, even in trace amounts, may interfere with hormonal balance, potentially disrupting metabolism and contributing to toxin buildup.

The presence of these contaminants in water adds to the body's toxic load, creating more work for detox organs like the liver and kidneys. Drinking contaminated water on a regular basis may gradually accumulate these toxins, affecting your health and undermining detox efforts.

Fortunately, there are several ways to ensure you're drinking the cleanest possible water and minimizing exposure to these contaminants. Here are some safer alternatives and methods to improve water quality:

Reverse Osmosis (RO) Reverse osmosis is one of the most effective filtration methods available. An RO system works by forcing water through a semipermeable membrane, which removes a wide range of contaminants, including heavy metals, chemicals, and microorganisms. RO systems are typically installed under sinks or as whole-house systems, providing a consistent supply of purified water. Many RO systems remove over 99% of impurities, making them a reliable choice for clean water. However, RO systems also remove beneficial minerals from water, so consider using a remineralization cartridge to add minerals back into your water.

Activated Carbon Filters Activated carbon filters are a more affordable and convenient option. These filters work by attracting and trapping impurities, particularly chlorine, volatile organic compounds (VOCs), and some heavy metals. Carbon filters are often available as faucet attachments, countertop units, or pitcher-style filters. While activated carbon doesn't remove all contaminants, it can effectively reduce the level of many common chemicals and improve taste. High-quality carbon filters may also reduce microplastics in water.

Distillation Distillation systems purify water by boiling it, capturing the steam, and condensing it back into liquid form. This process removes a wide range of contaminants, including heavy metals, fluoride, and most chemicals. However, like reverse osmosis, distillation also removes beneficial minerals, so it's often best to add minerals back in or combine distilled water with other mineral sources.

BPA-Free and Stainless Steel Bottles If you're using bottled water or carrying water on the go, opt for BPA-free plastic bottles or stainless steel bottles to minimize exposure to plastic chemicals like BPA and phthalates. BPA is a hormone disruptor that can leach into water, especially when exposed to heat, so using BPA-free or stainless steel options helps prevent additional toxic exposure. Stainless steel bottles are also more durable and eco-friendly.

Hydration is essential for lymphatic health, but water quality is just as important as quantity. Clean, contaminant-free water supports the lymphatic system by reducing the intake of harmful substances, easing the body's detoxification processes, and promoting optimal hydration. By choosing purer water sources and using safe, reusable bottles, you can reduce your toxic load, support efficient toxin elimination, and empower your lymphatic system to function at its best. This small investment in water quality can yield lasting benefits, enhancing both immediate wellness and long-term resilience.

Stimulating the Lymphatic System

The lymphatic system is a crucial part of the body's detoxification process. It removes toxins, waste products, and excess fluids from tissues, supports immune function, and helps maintain fluid balance. Unlike the circulatory system, which relies on the heart to pump blood, the lymphatic system doesn't have its own pump. Instead, lymph fluid moves through the body with the help of muscle movement, breathing, and other external factors. As a result, practices that stimulate lymph flow can play a significant role in detoxification, improving overall health and aiding in weight management.

In this chapter, we'll explore various methods for stimulating the lymphatic system, from self-lymphatic massage and exercise to dry brushing, hydrotherapy, and detox baths. Each technique supports lymph flow, helping the body eliminate toxins more effectively and promote wellness.

Lymphatic drainage massage, or lymphatic massage, is a gentle, therapeutic technique that encourages the natural movement of lymph fluids throughout the body. This practice supports the body's detoxification processes, helping to eliminate waste, reduce swelling, and enhance immune function. Performing self-lymphatic massage can offer relaxation, detoxification, and a boost in energy without requiring professional assistance, making it a powerful tool for your self-care routine:

Boosts Immune System By stimulating lymphatic flow, this massage helps cleanse the body of toxins and waste, supporting immune health and resilience against illness.

Reduces Swelling and Water Retention Lymphatic massage can be especially helpful for reducing puffiness and swelling, especially in the legs, arms, and face.

Promotes Relaxation and Stress Relief The gentle, rhythmic motions of lymphatic massage have a calming effect on the nervous system, providing mental relaxation and physical relief.

Supports Skin Health By improving circulation, lymphatic massage can help nourish skin cells, promoting a healthy glow and reducing blemishes and puffiness.

Creating a calming environment in which to perform your lymphatic drainage massage can help you relax, making the experience more effective and enjoyable. Here's how to prepare:

Find a quiet, peaceful area where you won't be disturbed. Dim the lights, play soft music, or light a scented candle to set a calming atmosphere that helps you focus on the massage and encourages relaxation. Keep the room warm enough to avoid feeling cold during the massage, as it will help your muscles and lymphatic vessels stay relaxed.

Use a light, unscented oil or lotion, like jojoba or almond oil, to reduce friction during the massage. A small amount goes a long way; you just want enough to help your hands glide smoothly over your skin.

Choose a comfortable chair, bed, or cushioned area where you can sit or lie down, allowing you to fully relax during the process.

Follow these instructions to perform a full-body lymphatic massage on yourself, focusing on the main lymphatic pathways. Remember that light, gentle pressure is key, as the lymphatic vessels are just below the skin's surface. Deep pressure can impede lymph flow, so aim for a soft, calming touch.

Begin with the Neck and Shoulders

Begin by placing your fingertips just below your ears. Use gentle, upward strokes, moving the skin in the direction of your lymph nodes (towards your collarbone). Light pressure and slow, rhythmic motions are most effective. Make small, circular movements from behind your ears, down the side of your neck, and toward your collarbone. This movement helps drain lymph fluid from the head and neck area to the lymph nodes located near your clavicle. Do this motion 5-10 times, focusing on creating a calm, rhythmic flow.

Massage the Arms

Place your opposite hand at your wrist, and use long, gentle strokes moving up towards your armpit. When you reach the armpit, apply a slight pumping motion. This action stimulates the lymph nodes located here, helping to activate the lymphatic system and support drainage. Work each section of the arm, moving from wrist to elbow, then elbow to shoulder, always in the direction of the armpit. Perform 5-7 strokes per section for effective results.

Focus on the Chest and Abdominal Area

Place your hands around the outer edges of your chest, near the armpits. Using soft, circular motions, gently massage inwards toward the underarm area where lymph nodes are concentrated. Avoid pressing directly over the breast tissue; instead, use light pressure around it.

Abdominal Area

Use gentle tapping or circular motions across your abdomen, starting from the lower belly and moving upward. The tapping motion can help stimulate lymphatic flow and support digestion. Move your hands from your sides towards the center of your torso, directing lymph toward the body's main drainage areas.

Breathe Deeply

Breathing deeply during abdominal massage can further support lymphatic flow and encourage relaxation. Inhale slowly, allowing your belly to rise, and exhale as you continue the massage.

Massage the Legs

Begin with your fingertips at your ankles and use smooth, upward strokes, moving towards your groin area.

Gently stroke from your ankles to your knees, then from your knees to your upper thighs, focusing on directing lymphatic fluid towards the pelvic region where lymph nodes are concentrated.

Knead Calves and Thighs

Use gentle kneading or circular motions on areas of the legs that feel tight or swollen. Focus on areas prone to fluid retention, such as the inner thighs and calves.

Perform 5-10 strokes per section, always moving upwards toward the core to promote lymphatic drainage.

ADDITIONAL TIPS FOR EFFECTIVE LYMPHATIC MASSAGE

Be Mindful of Pressure

Lymphatic massage requires only light pressure. Imagine the pressure you'd use to move the surface of a balloon without popping it. Going too deep can actually restrict lymphatic flow.

Work in Sections

Instead of trying to do a full-body massage all at once, focus on one area at a time. Give each section the attention it needs, allowing for slow, rhythmic strokes.

Deep Breathing

During your massage, incorporate deep breathing. Inhale deeply through your nose, allowing your abdomen to rise, and exhale slowly. Deep breathing naturally stimulates lymph flow and enhances relaxation.

Consistency is Key

Like any wellness practice, the benefits of lymphatic massage improve with consistency. Aim to perform self-lymphatic drainage two to three times a week for best results, especially if you experience swelling, sluggishness, or stress.

Self-lymphatic drainage isn't just about relaxation; it's a way to help your body process and eliminate waste more efficiently. By moving lymph fluid through your lymphatic system, you're reducing the buildup of waste and excess fluid that can lead to swelling, sluggishness, and a weakened immune system.

As the lymphatic system doesn't have a natural pump like the heart, it relies on movement and massage to push lymphatic fluid through the body. This helps remove toxins that would otherwise accumulate.

By increasing blood flow and supporting lymphatic function, this massage can lead to a clearer, healthier complexion by reducing puffiness and stimulating nutrient delivery to skin cells.

Also, lymphatic massage has a calming effect on the nervous system, providing a sense of relaxation and stress relief that can benefit mental health and promote restful sleep.

By integrating lymphatic drainage massage into your self-care routine, you're supporting both your body's detoxification and your overall wellness. This simple, mindful practice can have a profound impact on your energy, immunity, and sense of well-being.

Self-lymphatic massage can be a powerful tool for supporting your lymphatic system and overall health. When done consistently, it helps reduce swelling, boost immunity, and enhance detoxification.

Incorporating self-lymphatic drainage, especially when performed along with dry skin brushing can be transformative for your overall health.

DRY SKIN BRUSHING: A SIMPLE ROUTINE FOR HEALTHIER SKIN AND LYMPH FLOW

Dry brushing is a straightforward and effective technique that promotes exfoliation, improves circulation, and supports lymphatic drainage. Just a few minutes a day can help your body remove toxins and reveal smoother, more radiant skin.

Exfoliate Dead Skin Cells Dry brushing removes dead skin cells, leaving your skin feeling softer and looking brighter. Regular exfoliation helps prevent clogged pores, smooths rough patches, and promotes even skin texture.

Boosts Circulation The brushing motion encourages blood flow, which increases the delivery of oxygen and nutrients to the skin and underlying tissues, resulting in a healthy glow.

Stimulates Lymphatic Drainage Dry brushing helps stimulate lymph flow, supporting the removal of toxins and waste from the body. This process contributes to reduced swelling and improved immune function.

May Reduce the Appearance of Cellulite Many people find that dry brushing over time helps smooth out bumpy areas on the skin, particularly in areas prone to cellulite.

Improves Skin Texture Regular dry brushing helps skin become softer and smoother by continuously removing dead skin cells.

HOW TO PERFORM DRY SKIN BRUSHING

Choose the Right Brush Look for a natural-bristle brush with a firm yet gentle texture. A brush with a long handle is ideal, as it allows you to reach all areas of your body comfortably. You've undoubtedly seen these in the bath aisle at most major retailers, or on Amazon for about $10.

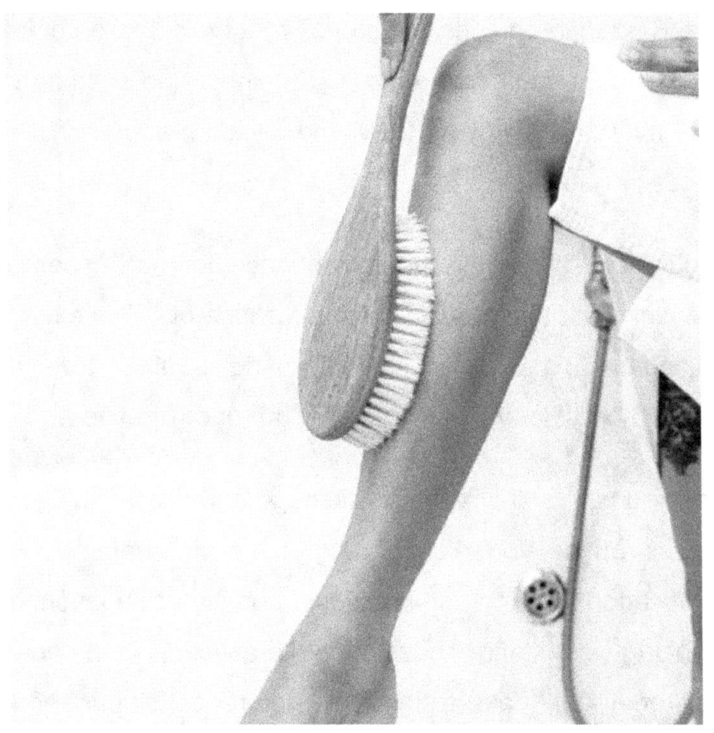

Best Time to Brush The ideal time to dry brush is before your shower. Brushing before showering allows you to wash away dead skin cells and impurities that have been loosened by the brush.

How to Dry Brush Start at your feet and brush upward toward your heart, using gentle strokes. Move from the legs to the arms, and then to the torso, always brushing in the direction of the heart. Be gentle on sensitive areas, and avoid broken or irritated skin. Brush 2 minutes up each leg, 2 minutes up each arm, and then 2 minutes down your torso and back, for a total of 10 minutes per session.

Regular dry brushing promotes lymphatic flow, enhances circulation, and can reduce the appearance of cellulite by breaking up fluid retention in tissues. Additionally, it exfoliates dead skin cells, leaving the skin smooth and refreshed.

By adding both self-lymphatic massage and dry brushing to your wellness routine, you're supporting your body's natural detoxification and immune functions, boosting circulation, and enhancing skin health. These simple practices, when done consistently, can make a significant difference in your energy levels, skin texture, and overall sense of well-being. Give it a try, and experience the transformative effects of these time-honored techniques.

Certain types of physical activity are particularly effective in promoting lymph flow and supporting detoxification. Here are some of the best exercises for stimulating the lymphatic system:

Rebounding and Vibration Plates Rebounding involves bouncing on a mini-trampoline, while vibration plates provide gentle whole-body vibrations. Both of these activities are effective for stimulating lymphatic circulation because they create a rhythmic, vertical motion that compresses and releases lymph vessels, helping push lymph fluid through the system.

Just 10–15 minutes on a mini-trampoline or vibration plate can improve lymphatic flow, increase circulation, and strengthen the immune system. Rebounding also helps tone muscles, supports balance, and is easy on the joints, making it accessible for most fitness levels.

Yoga and Pilates Yoga and Pilates are low-impact exercises that incorporate deep breathing, stretching, and controlled movements, all of which support lymphatic flow.

Poses such as Sun Salutation, Downward Dog, Twists, and Legs-Up-the-Wall help reverse blood flow, compress and release tissues, and stimulate lymph nodes. The breathing techniques used in yoga also encourage lymph movement and promote relaxation, which helps reduce stress-related inflammation.

Pilates involves controlled movements that engage core muscles and improve circulation. Many Pilates exercises involve lifting the legs or engaging the abdomen, which compresses the lymph nodes in the abdominal area and encourages lymphatic drainage.

Walking and Swimming Simple forms of cardio, like walking and swimming, are also excellent for lymphatic health. Regular walking is one of the easiest and most effective ways to keep lymph fluid moving. As your leg muscles contract and relax with each step, they gently push lymph fluid toward the lymph nodes. Aim for at least 30 minutes of brisk walking each day to support lymphatic flow.

The horizontal position of swimming, combined with water pressure, naturally stimulates lymphatic flow. Swimming also engages the entire body, providing a gentle yet effective form of resistance exercise that improves circulation and aids in detox.

Hydrotherapy Hydrotherapy, or water therapy, involves alternating between hot and cold water to stimulate circulation and lymphatic flow.

Contrast Showers To perform a contrast shower, alternate between 1-2 minutes of warm water and 30 seconds of cold water, repeating this cycle several times. The sudden change in temperature causes blood vessels and lymph vessels to constrict and dilate, which encourages lymph movement.

Hot Baths and Cold Rinses Soak in a hot bath for a few minutes, then briefly rinse with cold water. This can be done at the end of a shower or as a standalone treatment.

DETOX BATHS

Detox baths are another effective way to support the lymphatic system and enhance detoxification. These baths involve adding natural ingredients to the bathwater that help draw out toxins, relax muscles, and reduce inflammation.

Epsom Salt Bath Epsom salt is rich in magnesium sulfate, a mineral that relaxes muscles, reduces inflammation, and draws toxins out of the body through the skin. Add 1-2 cups of Epsom salt to a warm bath and soak for 20–30 minutes. Epsom salt baths can help relieve muscle tension, promote relaxation, and encourage lymph flow.

Apple Cider Vinegar Bath Apple cider vinegar has natural detoxifying properties and helps balance the skin's pH, which is beneficial for the skin's natural barrier function. Add 1-2 cups of raw apple cider vinegar to a warm bath and soak for 20–30 minutes. Apple cider vinegar baths can be soothing for irritated skin and may help support lymphatic detox.

Essential Oils Adding essential oils like lavender, eucalyptus, or juniper can enhance the detox benefits of your bath and provide additional lymphatic support. Add a few drops of essential oil to your bath, or dilute the oil in a carrier oil before adding it to prevent skin irritation. Be careful not to add more than a few drops because the oils may cause a burning sensation.

Bentonite Clay Bath Bentonite clay is a powerful natural detoxifier that helps draw out impurities, heavy metals, and toxins from the body. To use it in a detox bath, add about 1/4 to 1/2 cup of bentonite clay to warm bath water, mixing it in well to avoid clumps. Soak for 20–30 minutes to allow the clay to absorb toxins through the skin, promoting a deep, purifying experience that can leave you feeling refreshed and rejuvenated.

Herbs and Adaptogens for Detox

The lymphatic system is one of the body's primary detox pathways, and certain herbs and adaptogens are powerful natural allies in supporting the body's detoxification processes. While some herbs specifically stimulate lymph flow, helping the body clear toxins through the lymphatic system, adaptogens work at a deeper cellular level to enhance resilience to stress, promote cellular repair, and support overall health. Additionally, natural detoxifying agents like castor oil and apple cider vinegar offer unique benefits for enhancing detoxification, both externally and internally.

Here are a few potent lymph-stimulating herbs to consider:

Red Clover Red clover is well-known for its blood-purifying properties and its ability to improve lymphatic circulation. This herb contains phytoestrogens, antioxidants, and anti-inflammatory compounds, making it beneficial for overall detoxification.

Red clover helps thin lymph fluid, allowing it to flow more freely through lymphatic vessels and be filtered efficiently. Its anti-inflammatory properties support the lymphatic system, reduce congestion, and promote the elimination of waste.

How to Use Red clover is commonly consumed as a tea. Steep 1-2 teaspoons of dried red clover flowers in hot water for 10–15 minutes. Drink 1-2 cups per day to support lymphatic health. It's also available in tincture form, which can be added to water or juice.

Cleavers Cleavers, also known as "sticky weed," is one of the best herbs for supporting lymphatic drainage. It is a gentle diuretic, meaning it encourages the removal of excess fluids, which can reduce swelling and help the body eliminate toxins.

Cleavers promotes lymphatic movement and detoxification by stimulating lymph flow and assisting the kidneys in flushing out waste. It's particularly helpful for reducing fluid retention and lymphatic congestion.

How to Use Cleavers can be made into a tea by steeping 1–2 teaspoons of dried herb in hot water for 10 minutes. For a more concentrated option, cleavers tincture can be taken by adding 1-2 droppers to water once or twice daily. Fresh cleavers can also be juiced and added to green smoothies for an extra detox boost.

Dandelion Dandelion is a powerhouse detox herb that supports both the liver and the lymphatic system. It has diuretic properties, helping the body release excess fluids and flush out toxins, while also aiding liver detoxification.

Dandelion supports lymph flow by reducing fluid retention and assisting the liver in processing and eliminating toxins. It also has anti-inflammatory properties that soothe the lymphatic system and aid in the removal of waste.

How to Use Dandelion root tea is a popular way to consume this herb. Steep 1–2 teaspoons of dried dandelion root in hot water for 15–20 minutes, and drink 1-2 cups daily. Dandelion is also available as a tincture or in capsule form.

These lymph-stimulating herbs, when taken consistently, can be a gentle and effective way to support lymphatic flow, reduce fluid retention, and promote overall detoxification.

Adaptogens are a unique class of herbs that help the body adapt to stress and support overall resilience. They don't directly stimulate lymph flow, but they work at a cellular level, promoting cellular repair and encouraging autophagy (the process by which cells "clean up" damaged components). Adaptogens are excellent additions to a detox program because they support long-term health, enhance the body's natural detox capabilities, and reduce the negative effects of stress, which can otherwise hinder detox efforts.

Ginseng Ginseng is known for its energizing and immune-boosting properties. It supports mental clarity, physical endurance, and resilience to stress, making it ideal for those seeking to improve vitality during a detox.

Ginseng has antioxidant properties that help protect cells from damage, supporting cellular health and potentially promoting autophagy. It also reduces inflammation and promotes mitochondrial function, which is essential for energy production and cellular detoxification.

How to Use Ginseng is available as a tea, tincture, or capsule. For tea, steep 1 teaspoon of dried ginseng root in hot water for

5–10 minutes, and drink up to two cups daily. Ginseng supplements are also available, though dosage may vary depending on the type (Asian vs. American ginseng), so it's best to follow product guidelines.

Ashwagandha Ashwagandha is a well-known adaptogen that reduces stress, balances hormones, and improves mood. By lowering cortisol (a stress hormone), ashwagandha allows the body to focus on detox and cellular repair.

Ashwagandha's ability to lower cortisol indirectly supports detoxification by reducing stress-related inflammation and promoting autophagy. It also has antioxidant properties that protect cells from oxidative damage.

How to Use Ashwagandha is commonly taken in capsule or powder form. For powders, mix 1/2–1 teaspoon into water, smoothies, or tea once daily. It's also available as a tincture, which can be added to water or juice.

Rhodiola Rhodiola is an adaptogen that fights fatigue, improves mental clarity, and enhances physical stamina. It's particularly useful for combating the effects of stress on the body and supporting a clear mind during a detox.

Rhodiola promotes cellular health by reducing inflammation and protecting cells from oxidative stress, which is essential for detoxification. It also stimulates autophagy, helping to clear damaged cellular components and promoting longevity.

How to Use Rhodiola is usually taken in capsule or tincture form. A typical dosage is 100–200 mg of rhodiola extract daily. Follow product instructions, and take it in the morning to prevent interference with sleep.

Incorporating adaptogens like ginseng, ashwagandha, and rhodiola into a detox regimen can help enhance the body's stress resilience, support cellular health, and encourage a state of calm that is conducive to healing and detoxification.

USING CASTOR OIL AND APPLE CIDER VINEGAR FOR DETOX

Castor oil and apple cider vinegar (ACV) are two natural substances with powerful detox benefits. They can be used internally and externally to support lymphatic drainage, improve digestion, and encourage the elimination of toxins.

Castor Oil Castor oil is known for its ability to stimulate lymph flow, improve digestion, and reduce inflammation. When applied externally, it can increase lymphatic circulation and support detoxification through the skin.

Castor oil contains ricinoleic acid, a fatty acid with anti-inflammatory and analgesic properties. When applied as a castor oil pack on the skin, it enhances circulation and stimulates lymph flow in underlying tissues, helping to clear toxins from the body.

How to Use: To make a castor oil pack, saturate a cloth in castor oil and place it over your abdomen or the area of concern (such as the liver). Cover with plastic wrap, place a hot water bottle or heating pad over it, and let it sit for 30–60 minutes. Castor oil packs can be done 2–3 times per week to stimulate lymph flow and support detox.

Apple Cider Vinegar (ACV) ACV is rich in acetic acid, enzymes, and beneficial bacteria, which support digestion, balance pH levels, and encourage detoxification. It can be consumed internally or used in detox baths for an external cleansing effect. Internally, ACV stimulates digestive enzymes, improves gut health, and helps the liver break down toxins more effectively.

How to Use Internally Mix 1–2 tablespoons of raw, unfiltered apple cider vinegar with a glass of water, and drink once daily before meals to improve digestion and support detox.

Both castor oil and apple cider vinegar are versatile tools in a detox regimen. Used regularly, they can help stimulate the lymphatic system, support liver function, and encourage the body to eliminate toxins more effectively.

Managing Stress and Emotional Toxins

When we talk about detox, we often think about eliminating physical toxins from food, water, and the environment. But emotional and mental toxins, such as chronic stress, negative thought patterns, and toxic relationships, can be just as harmful to our health. These emotional stressors affect our body in profound ways, influencing everything from our hormonal balance to our ability to lose weight and detoxify efficiently.

Stress is more than just a mental or emotional burden; it has real physical consequences. When we experience stress, our body releases cortisol, a hormone that helps us respond to stressful situations. But when stress is chronic—meaning it's constant or prolonged—cortisol levels can remain elevated, leading to several issues:

Cortisol and Detox Pathways High cortisol levels can slow down detoxification pathways in the liver, which is our primary detox organ. When these pathways are impaired, the body struggles to eliminate toxins efficiently, leading to a buildup that can affect overall health.

Cortisol and Weight Gain Chronic stress and elevated cortisol can also cause the body to store more fat, especially in the abdominal area. This is partly because cortisol increases cravings for high-sugar, high-fat foods, leading to overeating. Additionally, cortisol signals the body to conserve energy (store fat) rather than burn it, making weight loss more challenging.

In other words, managing stress is essential for effective detox and weight loss. Reducing cortisol can help support the body's natural detox processes and make it easier to reach and maintain a healthy weight.

Emotional toxins are just as real as physical toxins. Toxic relationships—whether with friends, family, or coworkers—can have a significant impact on our health. Here's how they affect us:

When we're around people who drain our energy, criticize us, or constantly bring negativity, our bodies react as if we're under threat, releasing stress hormones like cortisol. Over time, these emotional toxins can lead to the same issues as chronic stress: inflammation, digestive issues, weakened immunity, and hormonal imbalances.

Identifying and setting boundaries in toxic relationships is a powerful step toward emotional detox. This can be challenging, but it's essential for creating a healthier environment for yourself. Taking time to evaluate relationships, communicate your needs, and, if necessary, distance yourself from negative influences can have a tremendous impact on both mental and physical health.

Mind-body practices are powerful tools for managing stress, clearing emotional toxins, and supporting overall well-being.

Meditation involves focusing your mind and achieving a state of calm and clarity. Regular meditation has been shown to reduce cortisol levels, improve focus, and increase emotional resilience. By helping the body shift out of "fight or flight" mode, meditation supports the body's natural detox pathways and helps prevent stress from taking a physical toll.

Mindfulness is the practice of being fully present in the moment, noticing your thoughts and feelings without judgment. Mindfulness helps reduce rumination, or the tendency to dwell on negative thoughts, which can be a major source of emotional stress. Practicing mindfulness can help you become more aware of your triggers and handle stressors more calmly.

Breathwork involves intentional breathing exercises that activate the body's relaxation response. Techniques like deep belly breathing, box breathing, or alternate nostril breathing can reduce cortisol levels almost instantly, signaling the body to relax. By incorporating breathwork into your daily routine, you can help reduce the physiological effects of stress and promote a sense of calm and well-being.

By addressing stress, emotional toxins, and implementing mind-body practices, we can create a healthier internal environment that supports detoxification, weight management, and overall health. Managing stress and emotional toxins isn't just about feeling better mentally—it has real, tangible effects on physical health and our body's ability to detox. Taking steps to reduce stress, set boundaries in relationships, and practice mindfulness is a holistic approach that can make a big difference in your journey toward a healthier, toxin-free life.

Healing Inflammation With Electrons from the Earth

Grounding, or "earthing," is the practice of physically connecting with the Earth by walking, standing, or sitting barefoot on natural surfaces like grass, sand, soil, or water. This practice is based on the idea that the Earth's surface carries a subtle negative electric charge, and direct contact with it allows our bodies to absorb these electrons. By restoring this natural electrical connection, grounding may help balance the body's internal electrical state, reduce inflammation, and support cellular energy production.

The Role of ATP in Cellular Health and Inflammation At the cellular level, the body's primary source of energy is adenosine triphosphate (ATP), a molecule that powers nearly every cellular function. ATP production occurs in the mitochondria, where nutrients and oxygen are converted into energy that fuels cells. However, inflammation and oxidative stress can interfere with this process by damaging mitochondria, which limits ATP production and leaves cells less capable of performing vital functions, including repair and immune responses.

Research suggests that grounding may improve ATP production by reducing oxidative stress and inflammation, which can help protect mitochondria and support more efficient energy production. When we ground, the Earth's electrons can neutralize excess free radicals in the body, reducing oxidative damage and allowing mitochondria to function optimally. This boost in ATP levels is particularly valuable for healing and recovery, as it gives cells the energy they need to repair tissues and maintain overall health.

HEALTH BENEFITS OF GROUNDING FOR REDUCING INFLAMMATION AND BOOSTING ENERGY

Reduced Pain and Swelling Grounding has been shown to reduce pain, stiffness, and swelling, especially for those dealing with chronic inflammatory conditions. By reducing oxidative stress, grounding may help protect mitochondria and preserve ATP production, which supports healing and reduces discomfort in inflamed tissues.

Enhanced Immune Response Chronic inflammation can weaken the immune system over time. Grounding helps regulate this response by reducing oxidative stress, allowing the immune system to operate more efficiently. Improved ATP production also provides immune cells with the energy they need to fight infections and repair tissue damage effectively.

Improved Sleep and Reduced Stress Inflammation can worsen with chronic stress and poor sleep. Grounding has been shown to improve sleep quality and reduce stress by balancing cortisol, the body's main stress hormone. When stress levels decrease, the body can focus on healing and regenerating ATP, leading to better overall energy and resilience against inflammation.

Better Circulation Grounding has been linked to improved blood flow, which enhances oxygen and nutrient delivery to cells. By supporting optimal blood flow, grounding helps ensure that mitochondria receive the resources needed for ATP production, reducing inflammation and accelerating recovery.

Using Grounding Products Indoors For those who may not have easy access to outdoor grounding, grounding technology offers a convenient way to bring these benefits indoors. Grounding products, such as grounding mattress pads and sheets, are designed to connect you to the Earth's energy through your home's electrical system. These products contain conductive fibers that plug into the grounding port (third prong) of a standard electrical outlet, which is connected to the Earth outside. This setup allows electrons to flow from the Earth into your body, supporting grounding and ATP production while you sleep or rest.

How to Use Grounding Mattress Pads and Sheets

Grounding Mattress Pads Place a grounding mattress pad on your bed, either underneath or on top of your regular sheet, and connect the cord to the grounding port in a nearby outlet. This setup allows your body to receive grounding benefits, like reduced inflammation and improved cellular energy, throughout the night.

Grounding Sheets Similar to mattress pads, grounding sheets have conductive fibers woven into the fabric. Place them on your bed and connect them to the grounding port. Sleeping on a grounding sheet provides continuous grounding exposure, which may help regulate inflammation, support ATP production, and improve sleep quality.

Safety and Precautions Before using any grounding product, verify that your outlet is properly grounded with a grounding tester (available at most hardware stores). Follow manufacturer instructions to ensure safe and effective grounding.

How to Incorporate Grounding into Your Daily Routine

Combining outdoor grounding with grounding products can maximize benefits. Here are a few ways to get started:

Walk Barefoot Outside Spend 10-20 minutes walking barefoot on grass, sand, or soil, allowing your body to absorb the Earth's electrons, which may reduce inflammation and support ATP production.

Sit or Lie on Natural Surfaces If walking isn't an option, simply sit or lie down on the ground in a natural setting, even placing your hands or feet on the Earth for an energy boost.

Use Grounding Products Indoors Incorporate grounding products like mattress pads or sheets to ensure daily grounding exposure. These tools are ideal for those with limited outdoor access or in colder climates, providing consistent benefits for inflammation and cellular energy.

Grounding is a natural and accessible way to support the body's healing processes. By connecting with the Earth, whether through direct contact or grounding technology, we can reduce oxidative stress, balance inflammation, and enhance ATP production for optimal cellular function. Grounding may be particularly beneficial for those managing chronic pain, fatigue, or inflammation, as it promotes mitochondrial health, providing the energy needed for cellular repair and resilience. Embracing grounding as part of a daily routine can offer a gentle yet powerful path to improved well-being, making it easier to maintain a balanced, healthy life. For more information on how grounding works, watch The Earthing Movie by Rebecca and Josh Trickell (documentary on YouTube).

The Power of Intention in Detox and Healing

When we think about detoxing and healing, we often focus on physical actions: eating healthier, drinking more water, exercising, and using specific detox methods. However, the mind and body are deeply connected, and our thoughts, beliefs, and intentions play a significant role in how effectively we can heal and restore balance.

The saying "mind over matter" isn't just a cliché; it's rooted in science. Research has shown that our thoughts and intentions can impact our physical health through the mind-body connection. Here's how:

The Power of the Placebo Effect

The placebo effect illustrates that when people believe they are receiving treatment—even if it's just a sugar pill—they often experience real health improvements. This demonstrates that our beliefs and expectations can influence physical outcomes, highlighting the mind's power in the healing process.

Stress, Positive Thinking, and Detox

Chronic negative thinking and stress trigger the release of stress hormones like cortisol, which can disrupt the body's detox pathways, weaken the immune system, and slow down healing. In contrast, positive thinking and setting clear intentions reduce stress levels, helping the body function in a more balanced and relaxed state. This shift allows detox organs—such as the liver, kidneys, and lymphatic system—to work more effectively.

Setting Intentions for Detox and Healing

Setting an intention gives the mind direction and purpose. Rather than simply going through the motions, intentions focus your energy on a specific goal. For example, if your intention is to support your body's natural detox, you might affirm, "I am releasing what no longer serves my body and mind." This type of affirmation fosters a positive mindset that reinforces every healthy choice you make, from the foods you eat to how you manage stress.

Visualization is a powerful technique that involves using your imagination to picture yourself reaching your health goals. This isn't just daydreaming; visualization helps the brain practice what it feels like to achieve a goal, reinforcing motivation and commitment. Here's how visualization can support detox and weight loss:

The Brain Can't Distinguish Between Real and Imagined Experiences Studies have shown that the brain processes imagined experiences similarly to real ones. When you visualize a positive outcome—like a cleaner, healthier body—you engage parts of the brain involved in motivation and focus. This helps you stay committed to your detox or weight loss journey, as you're continuously "practicing" success in your mind.

Visualizing Toxins Leaving Your Body During a detox, try visualizing the toxins being released and eliminated from your body. Picture each breath, sweat, or sip of water helping to cleanse and refresh your system. This visualization can reinforce the idea that every positive action you take—whether it's drinking water, eating a healthy meal, or getting a good night's sleep—is contributing to your body's detox process.

Focusing on Weight Loss Goals If weight loss is part of your detox journey, visualization can be especially effective. Picture yourself feeling lighter, healthier, and full of energy. Imagine the small but meaningful steps you're taking, like choosing healthier foods, moving your body, or saying no to processed foods, and see how each choice brings you closer to your goal. The mental reinforcement can make these choices feel more natural and aligned with your true intentions.

A positive environment—both internal and external—is essential for successful detox and healing. Here's how to cultivate the right mindset and supportive community around you:

Nurturing Self-Compassion and Patience Detoxing and healing take time, and the process is often not linear. Instead of focusing on quick results, embrace patience and self-compassion. Remind yourself that each step, no matter how small, is part of a larger journey toward health. Self-compassion helps reduce self-criticism, which can lower stress and make it easier to stay committed to your goals.

Creating a Supportive Environment Surround yourself with people who encourage and uplift you on your journey. Whether it's family, friends, or an online community, having a support system that shares your health goals can provide motivation, accountability, and emotional support. You might even consider joining a detox or health-focused group where members share tips, celebrate progress, and provide encouragement.

Clearing Out Negativity Just as you detox physically, you can also detox emotionally and mentally by reducing negative influences. This might mean limiting time with people who drain your energy, letting go of self-doubt, or reducing exposure to media that fuels anxiety or stress. By creating an environment that feels safe and positive, you'll naturally feel more inspired and empowered to continue making healthy choices.

Daily Affirmations and Positive Reminders To reinforce your intentions, try using daily affirmations that align with your goals. Simple phrases like "I am committed to my health," "I am creating a balanced and toxin-free body," or "I am deserving of a vibrant life" can help solidify your focus and keep you motivated. Consider placing these affirmations in visible areas, like your bathroom mirror or workspace, to serve as a constant reminder.

In summary, the power of intention in detox and healing is not just about physical actions but also about nurturing a mindset that supports transformation. By practicing positive thinking, setting clear intentions, visualizing success, and building a supportive environment, you create the ideal conditions for your body and mind to thrive. This holistic approach can help make your detox journey not only more effective but also more fulfilling and deeply transformative. Embrace the power of your thoughts, your intentions, and the community around you, knowing that you are actively participating in creating a healthier, balanced life.

Embracing a Lifestyle of Balance and Wellness

Detoxing isn't just a one-time event; it's a way to support your body over the long term. Embracing a lifestyle of balance and wellness means adopting sustainable practices that help maintain your health, manage weight, and boost your vitality in a natural and lasting way. In this section, we'll explore how to make detox a regular part of your routine, develop supportive daily habits, and embrace the holistic approach to wellness.

After an initial detox, it's essential to maintain the positive effects by incorporating detox-friendly habits into your everyday life. Long-term maintenance is about building a lifestyle that naturally supports your body's detox processes. Here's how you can approach it:

Incorporate foods that naturally support detoxification, such as leafy greens, cruciferous vegetables (like broccoli and cauliflower), and fiber-rich fruits, into your daily diet. These foods help cleanse the liver, support digestive health, and keep your energy levels stable. By making these foods a regular part of your meals, you continuously support your body's detox pathways.

Water is essential for nearly every bodily function, including the elimination of toxins. Commit to using the cleanest water possible and drinking enough water each day to stay well-hydrated, which aids in kidney function and supports clear, glowing skin. Herbal teas and lemon water are great additions to help promote gentle detoxification and support digestion.

Intermittent fasting is an effective long-term strategy that can help manage weight and support cellular repair through autophagy (a natural process where the body clears out damaged cells). By integrating fasting windows, such as 12 to 16 hours overnight, you give your body time to rest, digest, and reset, supporting a balanced metabolism and continuous detoxification.

Quality sleep is one of the most powerful (and often overlooked) aspects of detox and overall health. While you sleep, your body performs critical detox processes, including brain detoxification through the glymphatic system. Aim for 7-9 hours of restful sleep per night to support mental clarity, immune function, and balanced hormones.

Long-term maintenance isn't about perfection; it's about consistency and making small, sustainable choices that support your health and vitality over time. Creating a daily routine that supports detox and wellness is key to making these practices sustainable and enjoyable.

Start Your Day with Intention Beginning your morning with intention sets a positive tone for the day. Consider starting each day with a few minutes of mindful breathing, meditation, or an affirmation like "I am committed to my health and balance." This simple practice can help ground you and reduce stress, creating a mindset that's focused on well-being.

Daily Movement for Detox and Energy Regular movement is essential for keeping the lymphatic system flowing, aiding digestion, and boosting mood. Incorporate gentle, detox-supportive exercises such as walking, yoga, or stretching into your daily routine. Aim to move for at least 20-30 minutes a day, as even light exercise can stimulate circulation and promote the release of toxins through sweat.

Nourishing Self-Care Practices Self-care isn't just about pampering yourself; it's about giving your body what it needs to thrive. This can include practices like dry brushing (which stimulates lymphatic flow), Epsom salt baths (which help relax muscles and draw out toxins), and taking time to enjoy nourishing meals. These practices support both body and mind, making you feel more balanced and empowered.

Creating Consistency with Small, Doable Steps Consistency is key to making any habit stick. Rather than overhauling your entire lifestyle all at once, focus on small steps you can sustain. For instance, you might start by drinking an extra glass of water each day, adding a green vegetable to your meals, or dedicating five minutes each morning to mindfulness. Over time, these small habits will add up, creating a supportive routine that doesn't feel like a chore.

Setting Realistic Goals and Celebrating Progress Staying motivated can be challenging, especially when adopting new habits. Set realistic goals for yourself, and celebrate each milestone along the way. For example, if your goal is to drink eight glasses of water a day or avoid processed foods, recognize and reward yourself when you achieve these small wins. This keeps you motivated and focused on building a lifestyle that feels rewarding and achievable.

Detox is so much more than a cleanse or a quick fix. It's about creating a balanced life that empowers your body, mind, and spirit to thrive. By embracing a holistic approach, you recognize that detoxing isn't just about what you put into your body or take out—it's about supporting every part of yourself in a way that leads to greater resilience, joy, and long-term health.

Physical health, mental well-being, and emotional balance are all interconnected. By nurturing each of these areas, you build a foundation for overall wellness. Detoxing your body can improve your mood; reducing stress can support your immune system; eating well can sharpen your focus. Embracing the holistic approach means understanding that every small step you take toward health has ripple effects on your entire life.

Life will always have challenges, whether it's environmental toxins, stressful situations, or unexpected health issues. By adopting regular detox and wellness practices, you strengthen your body's natural defenses, so you're better equipped to handle whatever comes your way. This resilience isn't just physical—it's also mental and emotional, helping you navigate life's ups and downs with more balance and calm.

Finally, detoxing is about living in alignment with the best version of yourself. As you embrace a lifestyle of balance and wellness, you naturally begin to make choices that align with your intentions for health, whether that's prioritizing nourishing foods, taking time for self-care, or surrounding yourself with positive influences. This alignment creates a sense of fulfillment and empowerment, as you realize that every choice you make is a step toward your healthiest, happiest self.

In conclusion, by focusing on long-term maintenance, building a supportive daily routine, and embracing a holistic approach, you can integrate detox and wellness practices into your life in a meaningful way. This is about creating a lifestyle that doesn't feel restrictive but rather supportive, helping you live with energy, clarity, and resilience. Embrace this journey as an ongoing commitment to yourself, knowing that every effort you make contributes to a healthier, more balanced, and empowered life.